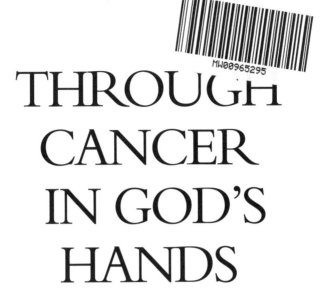

# THROUGH CANCER IN GOD'S HANDS

The Story of Ted and Mary Cornell

God wrote this book and I just delivered the message. I pray that you will hear His voice as you read it.

# TED CORNELL

IN GOD'S HANDS PUBLISHING CO.
1819 Pioneer Road
Shortsville, New York 14548-9205
ISBN 0-9721377-0-X

**Interlakes Oncology Hematology, P.C.**
I first met Ted and Mary Cornell in 1983. At the time, Ted had been diagnosed with small cell carcinoma of the lung, a disease which is rarely curable. Ted was treated on an investigational program, which consisted of chemotherapy, surgery and radiation therapy. The therapy was long and very difficult. Ted made it through this arduous journey with a combination of courage, determination, love and faith. Now 18 years after his diagnosis, Ted is obviously cured of his cancer and leading a full and active life.

In this little book, Ted and Mary document their journey towards cure. It should be an inspiration for anyone facing crisis in their lives, whether it be from cancer or some other factor.

*Robert F Asbury, md*

Robert F. Asbury, M.D.

Early in 1995 I was taking a bath and yelled out to Mary excitedly.

"What's the matter?", she asked.

"The Lord just told me we're going to write a book about my cancer," I said.

In order to write this book we had to go digging in the ashes caused by cancer. When you're digging you find live embers that begin to burn again, bringing back the pain of the past.

This is a story about love: love of a man for a woman, love of a woman for a man, love of both for their God. Through us may you see, in some measure, the reward that comes from loving a trustworthy God.

Introduction to Book
# Feelings Going Through Cancer

One of the first things we noticed was that the cancer was drawing us closer together. The reality was we both had it. I carried it in my body while Mary carried it in her heart. Believe me, I don't know which one was harder.

Mary seemed to think it hurt more and went through deeper feelings because it was in her heart. Our children were always on our minds. You think entirely different when you are given only two months to live. Material possessions seem worthless. The only thing of value is your relationship with God, your family, and your close friends. In order to ride the wave of emotion, you really have to put it in God's hands and know that He is the Anchor that holds. The people at Cancer Action had explained to me a whole series of emotions I would be going through, such as denial (why me?), and deep depression. I never had any of these, thank God.

We had agreed to wait and tell the children at home, instead of at the hospital. Riding home after hearing that Ted only had eight weeks to live and the children not knowing yet, Mary broke down emotionally, not caring about anything. Mary had her own problem trying to drive with tears that wouldn't stop flowing, but God got her home safely.

**Ted's cancer was discovered Oct. 14, 1983**
This type of cancer is Small Cell Carcinoma of the lung, also called Oat Cell Carcinoma. It accounts for about 14% of all lung cancer and is generally found in persons who are heavy cigarette smokers. I was smoking over

two packs a day. I quit in August 1974 and the cancer was found nine years, three months later.

In the book The Facts About Cancer (1981) we learned that only 25% of all people with cancer of the lung are operated on. Of those, only about 25% survive more than five years after the surgery. Oat Cell Cancer can not be removed surgically. The treatment is chemotherapy, where certain combinations of drugs greatly extend the lifespan of the Small Cell Carcinoma victim. There are five different kinds of lung cancer, the worst of which is small cells.

U. S. Cancer facts and figures for 1984 incidence estimated 139,000 new cases and the mortality rate estimated at 121,000 deaths. Survival beyond five years after diagnosis is about 9% of all lung cancer patients.

Twenty percent of all lung cancers are diagnosed early, in the "localized" stage. The survival rate for these patients jumps to 39%.

The diagnosis in my case, after all the tests and the biopsy, was Small Cell Oat Seed Cancer. From its original sight it gives off about a million seeds a day that go throughout the body and start new cancers. It also likes to go to the head. Usually by the time it is found it is too late, because of the seeds. My case was discovered after a car accident before I had found any signs of the disease. Because the seeds spread so rapidly; two months to live was diagnosed. They wanted to try an experimental program of extreme doses of chemotherapy to kill the cells on the outside, then perform surgery to remove the cancer, then a follow up of whole-brain radiation and two years of chemo-therapy to take care of any of the seeds that might be still floating around.

Across the country, 47 people participated in this experiment and Dr. Asbury believe's that I'm the only one still alive. Because of this diagnosis we started making funeral plans. Not that we planned on using them, but only a fool would deny the possibility. Mr. Cummings has been the family mortician for years and years. So after being given two months to live we decided to go to Watertown for a visit. This would be a way to help Mary. For a body to be transported from one county to another it has to be embalmed and we wanted to know if he could handle all the extra details. After our meeting was over he said it was harder on him than on us. We think it was due to his father's death from cancer. This is the way we planned and prepared day by day but we always kept long term goals as well. I have found this to be the best way. Long term and short term and always planning.

**God healed me**
Shortly after the diagnosis I started praying to God for a divine healing. Many people pray thusly because they don't want to go through the treatments and if they don't get healed they blame Him. He has an arsenal of weapons to use whether it is medicine or surgery; God controls it all. After all He performed His first surgery on Adam in Genesis. I prayed for divine healing, but if it was His will, I would go through this fire. Why do I call it a fire? Because it hurt like hell. They use chemotherapy and radiation; and its not like going on a picnic. When I hadn't been healed, I took the chemo praying that God would say, "That's enough." It wasn't, but before the next treatment they would do an x-ray to see how it was coming. I was praying that it would be

gone. And when it wasn't, I went through surgery, then radiation. This was to be followed up by two more years of chemotherapy and this is where God intervened. After two months of chemo my stomach became a problem that would have killed me if they had kept up with the chemo, so they had to stop. God said, "You've proved that you would go through the fire, so the next two years are on me."

# Introduction to Ted & Mary

When I read a book I like to know about the characters involved. So at this time I will introduce Ted and Mary. I was born Aug. 8, 1935, in Watertown, NY, one of four children of Grace and Henry Cornell. Henry was from Brooklyn, NY, and Grace from a little place called Clayton, NY. Mary was born on Wellesley Island, NY, about 35 miles from Watertown. She was the only child of Chancy and Ruth Patterson. Let's dwell for a minute on Chancy, known as the old decoy carver, who started carving at the age of fourteen and continued until 85 years of age, always doing it the same way. He passed away in our home at the age of 89.

Before going any further maybe we should tell you how we met. On March 17, 1954, Mary and I wound up at a dance in LaFargeville, NY, in between our two homes. I had just come back from Florida. Mary's Aunt Violet decided to go to the dance and asked Lillian, Joan and Sally if they wanted to go. Mary consented. I got my friend Gordy interested in going but neither one of us had wheels. So we went to another friend's house and he said he'd love to go but had no gas money, so we took care of that and away we went. When Mary looked up and saw me walking through the door she thought I'd make a good catch but she wouldn't be so lucky. But she was! After coming through the door, I was watching Mary dancing with Gordy. After his third dance with her, I said, "What's her name?"

He said, "I don't know."

I said, "You danced with that girl three times and you don't know her name? I'll dance with her once and I'll know all about her." I went over and asked her for a dance. Within four weeks we were talking marriage, but decided to wait because I was drafted in May of 1954 and discharged April of 1956. We were married Sept. 1, 1956. In July of 1957 our son came into the world. August 1960 our daughter joined our family, and the rest is history.

## Chapter One

# Introduction to Peg Leg
# First Man in the Room

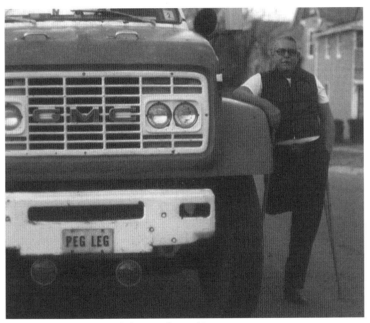

Peg Leg with his truck-his pride and joy.

In a story like this, where do you start? Since this is about cancer we will start at the point where I first came in contact with someone with it. He was a very close friend, named Peg Leg. He was a very unusual man. We lived near one another and rode together to work. Peg Leg had the reputation for being a very fast driver. A lot of the people at work would say, "How do you like riding on the white knuckle express?" I enjoyed it. It was quite a feat to see how that one foot would go from gas to brake; like watching an artist make a beautiful painting. Peg Leg lost his leg as a teenager and never wanted to be treated as an invalid. I never did, that's why we got along so well. But it caused a problem one day, when we were entering a restaurant and I was in front of him. He never wanted anyone to hold the door for him, so I didn't and he was closer than I thought. The door hit one of his crutches and down he went. I really felt badly. I turned to help him up and apologize, there he was laying on the floor looking up at me, laughing. He said, "I got just what I deserved for being so stubborn!"

Peg Leg also liked to drive tractor trailer. Probably the only person I know who could do such a feat with one leg. He earned the handle "Peg Leg" plugging through the mountains, meeting his schedules better than most. When highway officials discovered he only had one leg, they decided they were going to take his license. But he passed their driving test with his foot flying back and forth between the clutch, brake and gas pedals.

In the early spring of 1979, Peg Leg's wife called to notify us that he had cancer. That Easter Mary and I decided to go to the Hershey, PA hospital to visit him. When our close friends, Roland and Florence, heard the news they wanted to go along so we could all pray for him. On the way down to Hershey, as always going through PA., we had to stop at Mountain Top Diner. It had been a bit of a hangout for Peg Leg, and a natural stop for us anytime we headed south. On this particular day we pulled in and it was like pulling into home.

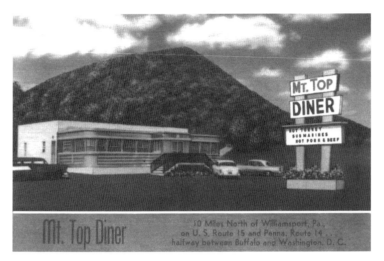

Mountain Top Diner; our home away from home. Peg Leg's hangout. We all loved it.

After lunch we sat with coffee and talked about Peg Leg, about how things might be when we arrive. We said a prayer that the news would be good. Back in the car and on to the hospital where we found out he had stomach cancer. We all prayed for him.

While our wives visited the hospital gift shop we talked together in the room. Peg Leg was smoking a cigarette and I commented on it. He said, "Nobody is going to tell me to quit now; for me it's too late." Then looking up from the bed he said, "You guys are lucky. They say one out of every three gets cancer and I'm the one. You two will escape it."

When he was dying, he said he had driven everything: cars, tractor trailers, motorcycles, bicycles, snow-mobiles, go karts, racing cars, anything with wheels. What he wanted to do now was to get in a big

13

airplane and at least taxi it. My son, who was in the Air Force at the time, was in the process of setting this up for him when Peg Leg passed on. He went where he didn't need a plane.

The day of the funeral Mary and I cried, realizing that this chapter of our life was over and we had to get over the loss of one of our closest friends. Thinking of how final cancer is, never again to meet him at Mountain Top, never again went on and on. How cruel cancer is! Now and again we cry with these memories.

*A true friend can cheer us in our sorrows,*
*Love us through our difficulties and failures.*
*There is nothing on this earth that is worth*
*More than a true friend.*
*Peg Leg fit it all.*

## Chapter Two

# Introduction to Roland
# Second Man in the Room

We met Roland and his wife at church and became close friends almost immediately. We'd plan dinners together and sit for hours talking about the Bible. Roland was not only a good Christian but he walked his talk. If we all had a good Christian friend like him, we could change the world. What an example! Roland owned a gas station and anytime you walked through the door you would hear sweet sounds of Christian music. His gas station almost felt like church. It was a place you could get your car fixed honestly, not being sold parts that weren't needed. You could feel that sweet, honest spirit in the place.

Once we went together to a Jimmy Swaggart Crusade in Buffalo, NY. After the crusade we decided to see if we could catch Jimmy before he got on his plane. As it turned out we rode out to his plane with him and he took us aboard to be introduced to the band members and his family. It was quite an experience for all of us.

We went on a few trips with Roland and his wife. One was to the Carolinas where we stopped at Carowinds Amusement Park. They have a roller coaster that goes from S. Carolina to N. Carolina and then back to S. Carolina. Roland wanted to go for one of those rides, but nobody wanted to chance it. Mary felt sorry for him but she was afraid. Roland promised to hold her hand so onto the roller coaster they went, waving good-bye to the chickens.

We took another trip to Florida and this time, one of his customers wanted to borrow his car for a couple of weeks. This gentleman had a Winebago camper. So he and Roland switched and the four of us packed up the Winebago and headed for Florida with the idea that we would see it all. We made it all the way down to Key West. We also were at Disney World for Christmas and then on to Miami for the New Years Parade. We took a ton of slides on this trip.

I have a little side story about these slides. Right after this trip Mary was scheduled for a hernia operation. While she was in the hospital we got the slides developed and decided to take them into the hospital with the projector and the table. The walls were white so we didn't need the screen. We got all set up, the four of us about to recapture our trip. But too much light was coming in from the hall, so we closed the door and the room was pitch dark. A little ways into the showing a nurse came busting through the door saying, "What is going on in here?" "We're watching slides from our trip" we told her. So she looked on the wall and saw these beautiful Florida pictures and she hollered out the door, "Come down here and see what's going on in this room!" The next thing we knew the room filled with people. We were the talk of the hospital.

The last trip we took with Roland was to Baton Rouge, Louisiana to a Jimmy Swaggart Crusade. Traveling on the way we passed Sammy Hall's bus. He was a popular gospel singer, I had several of his records in my collection. We had a CB radio and got on the air with Sammy's bus driver. Sammy was not on board. During our conversation I brought up a song that Sammy re-

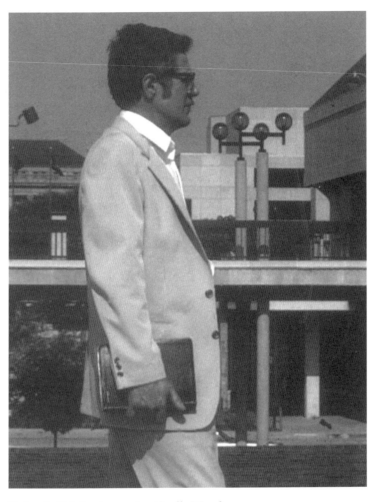

Roland at his best carrying God's Word.

corded called "Too Late." It is a very emotional song about being left behind after the Rapture of the church. At the time, CB's being very popular, many people were on the air talking back and forth. We played the song "Too Late" over the CB and you could not hear a word.

Everyone instead was listening to Sammy's song. There was a good three minutes of silence afterwards.

While on the road we started each day with a prayer and a devotional including a thought for the day. We then tried to apply that thought for the day. Each time we stopped we always placed a Bible tract in all the bathroom stalls so the people would have something to read.

While in Baton Rouge, Roland was driving and went off the road onto the shoulder a couple of times. We did not know it then but it was the beginning of melanoma cancer, which showed up as a mole on his chest that would bleed. We visited Roland a lot. We had called a number of Christian organizations to which he had donated large sums of money. We asked them to give Roland a call at this time, as he didn't have long to live. We knew what an inspiration this would be to him to hear from them. None of them called! We knew of one who was a preacher and a singer and Roland enjoyed listening to his music. His name was LaVerne Tripp. We told him of the situation and he immediately called Roland. What a blessing! He was not concerned with money; he was concerned for the soul. AMEN! Roland's wife called one day to say they didn't expect him to make it through the day. We stayed with him that day until he passed on. We made a special tape with Christian music that was played at the funeral home and at the service. One of the songs was "Gone."

When he died January 13, 1981, we had lost our closest Christian friend and it left our hearts grieving. He can't be replaced but we have our beautiful lasting memories. Roland had a very large library of Christian material such as books, tapes, and tracts. His wife gave this whole library to me. I thought how great this would be if anybody asks me a question about God or the Bible I'd have the answers. I had these materials for two or three years and had only a couple of questions to answer from them. I was reading a magazine about a place in India that was looking for Christian material. Realizing how much more they would get out of it, I started shipping to a place in Bihar Shariff, India. Later I came across an address for God's Children's Home in Ghana and I added this to my list. These places asked for clothes, kid's books, paper, pens, pencils, crayons and Bibles. We started going to garage sales and library sales. We kept right on shipping. In 1996 Ghana began having trouble with customs. They would hold the boxes we shipped and wanted fifty dollars to release them. The Home couldn't afford it, so we were asked to stop. But three or four years ago, they sent us a picture of forty or fifty children and not one had a pair of shoes on and four or five were just wrapped in a blanket. The last time they sent some pictures most were dressed and had shoes, thanks to the shipments.

The India people pray for us all the time. So do the people in Ghana. They pray we won't become ill or run out of funds, as they are in real need of our help.

So now you know the story of Roland's library. Some went to India, and some to Ghana, and it got us into the shipping business which we still do.

*A FRIEND IS SOMEONE WE TURN TO*
*WHEN OUR SPIRITS NEED A LIFT.*
*A FRIEND IS SOMEONE TO TREASURE*
*OUR FRIENDSHIP IS A GIFT.*
*A FRIEND IS SOMEONE WHO FILLS OUR LIVES*
*WITH BEAUTY, JOY AND GRACE.*
*AND MAKES THE WORLD WE LIVE IN*
*A BETTER AND HAPPIER PLACE.*

## Chapter Three

# My Trip through Cancer
# Third Man in the Room

I got my diagnosis two years later on October 14, 1983. Discovered in my lungs, it was called small cell oat-seed cancer. This type of cancer gives off almost a million seeds a day and spreads new cancer cells throughout the body. These small seeds like to go to the brain. Because of this type of cancer I was given two months to live. So much for Peg Leg's comforting statistic. Now, all three of us in the room had been diagnosed with cancer. Two are already dead, and I stand alone. Just a gentle reminder here that so far my contact with cancer had only been with death, and how cruel it is in the way that it affects the person and the family. I had certainly seen the devastating effects of it and felt them and still do.

We woke up in June 1983, to a normal day, not knowing that we had a date with destiny that would change our lives forever. Why do bad things happen to good people? I did not know it at the time, but a great tragedy would become a tremendous blessing. This accident was number one in a long string of blessings.

Our accident happened en route to Teen Challenge with a load of goods. Traveling on Interstate 490 at 55 miles an hour, Mary and I were rear-ended by someone who had been drinking. She had been traveling in excess of 100 miles an hour when our 1979 Cadillac got in her way.

Turns out, she was sitting in a bar in the middle of the afternoon until she remembered she had to pick up her mother. In a furious, foolish rush to meet her mother, she sped right up the road until her car struck ours. The girl's car came up over the rear bumper and into the trunk destroying the goods for Teen Challenge.

Our car careened off the highway, into a guard rail and almost over an embankment. Thank God for guard rails or we would have ended up on a set of railroad tracks. A few minutes later a train came through and we could have been in its deadly path. Praise God, we weren't.

When the young lady opened her car door a beer can rolled out. Immediately she approached Mary's side of the car wanting to drag her out and fight. She had no concern for our well being, only anger because she was late and we kept her from getting her mother on time.

The first car on the scene of the accident was someone we knew. This gentleman went and called our children and when he came back he brought coffee. We had witnessed to this gentleman a couple years prior. Johnny went through the Teen Challenge Program and had become a minister. He wrote a book, Even Me, which was about his life as a heroin addict. When we left the gentleman at the restaurant, where we witnessed to him, Johnny looked at him and said, "One thing from here on out, you'll never have the excuse you didn't know, because we just told you."

Our children picked us up after the accident and the car was towed away. They took us to look it over. It was a real sick looking puppy. We were reminiscing what a pretty car it was when we purchased it. What a sad ending. Although unknown to me at the time, that car

21

had just saved my life. If I had known it then I would have been more emotional. Thanks to God for this blessing!

Our insurance company put $8500 into the repair of our Cadillac. Blasted from behind and pounded front first into the guard rail, it needed a major overhaul. It's always been a thing with me, if anything major is done on an automobile, as soon as I can afford it, I trade it in. I've had a couple cars where I've had engines changed or transmissions and they'll be running good, but I'll trade them in because I've lost my faith in them. The 1979 Cadillac was no different. They had painted the whole outside and they put in a new transmission and it looked like it came off the showroom floor. I traded it in on my birthday, Aug. 8, 1983, and we bought a brand new 1983 Buick LaSabre. The story of the Cadillac continues. After I traded it in, the dealer found a problem so he wholesaled it out. A few months later I got a call from the police notifying me that they had my Cadillac. The guy who stole it was in jail and would I come down and sign the papers. I told them I had traded the car in a couple months ago and where I had traded it. It must have been stolen from the lot. I guess it was pretty well beat up. I don't know its final resting place. But God bless it, it helped save my life.

Another blessing occurred. When purchasing a new car we took out disability insurance. If I were to ever become sick, the insurance company would make the monthly payments on the loan - and they eventually did. When my pay was cut in half because of the cancer, we would not have been able to make the payments.

Because Mary and I were both hurting, we went to the hospital the day of the accident. The next day, after bleeding badly in the shower, Mary returned to the hospital. We spent two hours in the emergency room before being referred to a gynecologist.

After the accident, Mary was in and out of the hospital a few times and we were both going to a chiropractor. Dr. Schamberger, who was a Christian, prayed for us at each visit. Mary had bad whiplash.

I was placed on sick leave, because I had health problems all summer long. It was recommended that we go to our family doctor. Thank God my wife was the one that called. When she called the nurse to set up an appointment she checked our records finding we hadn't had physicals in 12 years. I was 48 at the time and had planned on having a complete physical at age 50. If I had waited I would have died before then. Thank God for God-fearing wives. Not paying any attention to me she set us up for a complete physical. The first thing was a lung x-ray in which they found a spot. Once they find a spot, they have to determine if there is mass to it. Therefore, a tomogram was scheduled.

When it was over, although not allowed to tell us then, I could read it on the face of the nurse. I knew I had cancer. I said to myself, "Now, it's my turn, the last of the three musketeers. The room will be empty." Knowing that my good Christian friend, Roland, didn't make it, I thought I'd never make it either. It's amazing the rambling thoughts that go through your mind at a time like this.

On October 26 the doctor called and confirmed what I had already figured out. When first diagnosed my mom was with us. She still was somewhat alert, but was coming down with Alzheimer's. We decided it best to take mom back to my brother Bob's house for a few months. It made it easier while going through the treatments. While she was there she told my brother that I would need a lounge chair and she wanted to buy it. They went shopping in Watertown and had it delivered through a Rochester store. It turned out that when they did the lung operation I couldn't lie down and be comfortable so I spent about a week sleeping in that chair. It seems amazing that while Alzheimer's was coming on she still had foresight and knew exactly what I would need, although I didn't. What a blessing a mother and a chair can be.

Immediately, the family started calling prayer requests to the following men and ministries: La Verne Tripp, the 700 Club, Jimmy Swaggart, Full Gospel Businessmen, Jack Van Impe and our church fellowship with Pastor Paul Colosi. Also, Pastor Jergen, who was involved in supporting Roland, came and stood with us in our crisis. His church in Chili was The Well and they prayed too.

Our old neighbors who became very, very close friends, were Ted and Paula. Paula was my very first inspiration after being diagnosed with cancer. She explained to me that she had a very unusual blood disease and that by rights she shouldn't be around. But if she could do it, I should be able to also. This is the kind of inspiration you need at a time like this.

Knowing there are a lot of ways to face cancer we thought about the options, Some people said because I am a good Christian I didn't have to worry about it, I don't have to go to a doctor. God will heal me. Other people told us the government doesn't know what it's doing, it is trying to sell me a bill of goods and their stuff will do me more harm than good. Others said the chemotherapy would kill me and if that doesn't the radiation will. Some Christians were telling me I had the devil in me or I wouldn't have cancer. There were people giving me all kinds of information, so I felt I had to sit down and figure it all out myself. I thought God had more than one way to heal, by divine intervention or by the doctor's hands.

To answer my Christian friends, I got out the Bible and started right in the beginning and figured I'd go through it until I found out whether the doctor should be involved. I only got to Genesis 2:21 where the Lord caused a deep sleep to fall upon Adam and he took one of his ribs and closed up the flesh in its place. It sounds like God performed the first operation. When I went into the hospital to have the operation the doctor caused a deep sleep to come upon me and I slept. He removed a rib, then the doctor took a part of my lung and closed up the flesh. One is God operating and the other is the doctor operating, but it is all the same.

The doctors get their abilities from God. One of the Apostles, Luke, also called the beloved physician, was a close friend and companion of Paul. If the only way to be healed was by divine intervention, then what was Luke doing? Healing is from God. The body has certain abilities to heal itself. For instance, a scab seals over a sore so it can heal itself and also rest. There are times when practical measures and helps are needed such as, medicine, doctors and surgeons to enable the body to restore health. There are also miraculous healings in which the power of God is experienced instantaneously. This is the kind of healing everyone hopes for, but God provides them all. Not everybody is going to receive miraculous healing. I know of people that have died because they wouldn't accept healing any other way except by a miracle. Maybe God up in heaven is looking down and saying, "Why will you not accept My healing in other ways? It's as if you want to tell Me what to do. Don't you know I provide it all, whether miraculous or otherwise?" It's all God.

# Chapter Four

# The Beginning of Cancer in our Lives

On Oct. 29 I had a postcard show and sale. Being Show Chairman for a couple of years, I was busy taking care of a lot of details. Mary and I collected 1000 Islands postcards because of where she was from. It was a natural choice. At the shows we put up display boards; we put one together on the 1000 Islands using postcards and a little information about the cards. Our display took second place.

As I mentioned before my mother, who was living with us at this particular time, was struggling with Alzheimer's disease, but she knew enough to know that there was something major going on and it bothered her a lot. So Mary and I thought it over and decided it best for her if we took her to my brother's house.

He took care of her summers and we had her winters. I knew for the rest of the winter it would have been very stressful for her at our place. When next fall came around she came back to stay with us. We had to come right back on the 2nd because my son was going to graduate from Kodak on Nov. 3rd. It is great to see your children improve themselves. One of his bosses came over and told us what a good man he was. A beautiful dinner was served before the ceremony. It brought tears to our eyes to see our son get his diploma, as he had served his apprentice ship for control systems.

On November 4th I had an appointment with Doctor Craver. He was the lung surgeon, and at this time we knew it was cancer but not what kind. He thought only a simple surgery would be needed. We set up a follow-up appointment for the 10th so they could do a lung biopsy.

While talking with the doctor I said, "I have a lot of faith in God to be healed. "Right away he asked if it was good faith or bad faith. This took me back as I had never heard of bad faith, so I said, "What do you mean by 'bad faith'?"

"You tell me your faith and I will tell you whether it's good or bad."

"I believe that God is the healer, whether He does it by divine intervention or by pills, by chemotherapy, radiation or your hands as a surgeon. He is the only one that can heal. But He does use all the other things including your hands."

"That is good faith," replied Doctor Craver. "Now I'll tell you a story of bad faith. I had a gentleman in the office in much the same position as you're in. I explained to him a treatment program and he said he didn't need it, God would heal him. All he had to do was go where there was a hill with about 150 steps and climb it on his knees saying prayers. He believed when he got to the top he would be healed. In order to finance the trip he sold his home and most of his possessions. He made that trip, climbed that hill, came back and died, leaving his wife and children penniless." So this proved to be bad faith, and my faith was considered to be good.

After that first appointment with Doctor Craver, we decided to take a break and try and get this off our minds. Cancer is not a very easy thing to wash off your mind, it just stays with you. We took a trip to Toronto on Nov. 5th to give it a try. When I got into the hotel room, for some reason, I went right to the window. Staring out across the city and thinking thoughts like, "Is there ever a winner?" "My friends both died, soon I'll be joining them." "Who am I, that I should expect anything different?" My thoughts were of heaven and life and what really matters. I stood like this for about an hour just gazing out the window. Mary allowed me to drift through my own thoughts while her mind told her things like feeling sorry for me and what if it was her? What was our life going to be like and how would it end? Then back to reality again and down the stairs we went. After all, this is Toronto, this is the Royal York and there is an underground shopping mall of 200 stores to be conquered. We walked all over that place, looking and longing, just wondering how many more weekends we might have together.

While still underground we walked back toward the hotel. Mary recalls a man approaching us and we started a conversation with him. After a short time, he asked what brought us to Toronto. We told him cancer, but he could not believe it. He asked how we could look so happy after being diagnosed with lung cancer? Our reply left him equally puzzled: God is on our side.

After the weekend, we traveled home through Tonawanda and spoke to Diane, Peg Leg's wife. It shocked her to know I too now had cancer. She could not believe it. Because she went through the loss of Peg Leg she wanted us to keep her posted about the progress of the disease. It brought us even closer. It is nice to know that we have people who are concerned for us. We talked over old times and the adventures we shared.

I went to work Nov. 8th and 9th but it was very difficult to get your mind on the job when you're thinking about cancer. The guys I worked with were very supportive and they tried to build up my spirit. The 10th was my biopsy. The day of truth. From this day on there would be no more guess work. Prior to this I could say maybe they misdiagnosed or maybe there was nothing there or maybe God healed me. So Mary and I planned on having lunch together after the appointment. It was not to be.

But God performed another blessing.

My biopsy required freezing the side of my torso and piercing through my ribs into my lungs to snatch a piece of cancerous tissue. The needle, equipped with a tiny camera-like device, plunged through my flesh probing and poking while I joined the doctors watching the video output on a monitor screen. Out came the sample for testing, which was rushed to the lab. They did not want the novocaine to wear off in case another sample was needed. I lay awake with a nurse standing by my side, watching over me.

As we waited I was beginning to see the room close in, so I asked the nurse if they had any special equipment available in case my lung went down. She said there was a special kit in the next room.

"It might be a good idea to get one, just in case," I said. She went out through a door, and when she returned a doctor came in right behind her. He wanted to know if she needed any help.

"No," she said, "he just wants to have the kit on standby."

By this time the room had closed in until I could just see a small portion of it. Then, Doctor Craver walked in and I said, "My lung is going down."

When your lung collapses they have to put a tube in your side to let the leaking air out of your chest area. In went the tube, sticking into me on one end and into a small water tank on the other end. Pushing this tube into my side was very painful, and from then on every movement or vibration sent a pain right through me making me cry. After the first few days, though, I got used to it, and there was no more pain.

When Mary walked in to check on me, she found me laying flat, crying because of the pain. This made her very emotional to see me this way. She could almost feel the pain. This was the most crying I had done through this whole cancer scenario.

That pain I can still feel today, but I am thankful for the collapsed lung, for they needed to admit me on November 10th for two weeks. This turned out to be a blessing from God. Had I remained an outpatient, I might have had lunch with Mary. Because I stayed, they came in at all hours, any hour, test after test after test, even late at night. Going through the halls lying on your back and everything quiet you think you're in the twilight zone, very eerie.

From the biopsy, my cancer diagnosis was small cell oat seed carcinoma.


**The next person that you'll be introduced to in this book is Katy, Joe's girlfriend, and what follows is how she felt during my time with cancer.**

During the latter part of 1983, I had occasion to be in the Pulmonary Care Unit at Genesee Hospital in Rochester, New York, visiting Joe McConnell, the man I was dating at the time. During that hospitalization, Joe and I had the pleasure of meeting another couple, Ted and Mary Cornell. They were close to our age and also going through a difficult time. Both men had life-threatening lung diseases, a dreadful fact that seemed to give them a common bond. Since both were there for an extended stay, we all became acquainted and made fast friends. To this day, I credit Ted's success in overcoming lung cancer not only to the aggressive oncological treatment he received, but also to his great faith in the Lord, his loving family support, and his ability to handle stress. Ted's family was constantly there for him - Mary, with her ever- present cheerful smile and bubbly demeanor, his son and his wife, and his daughter and her husband. Even their adorable granddaughter was there to cheer Grandpa. Her sweet, innocent, cherubic face would warm anyone's heart. What miraculous therapy this lovely family's affection and support provided!

Joe and I enjoyed some wonderful times with Ted and Mary over the next several years. In 1986, we moved to Florida, but have still kept in touch over the years. Through the grace of God, both men are still among us, still survivors. Since I am an oncology nurse, I'm always searching for ways to inspire my patients to keep the faith and keep a positive attitude. Over the last 14 years, I've used my friend Ted's story countless times as a source of inspiration for my patients. Imagine, being a lung cancer survivor for these many years! Just as in the 1946 classic, "It's a Wonderful Life," we seldom realize the far-reaching effects our solitary life can have. My dear friend, Ted, far away in New York State, has undoubtedly inspired people here in Daytona by his wonderful example of faith and perseverance.

## Chapter Five

# In the Hospital - Day to Day

On the first full day, Nov. 11th, I had a chest x-ray that morning and company that afternoon. My son-in-law, Bill, was there and I was complaining that my feet were cold. He went off somewhere and came back in about 10 minutes and had a nice warm blanket for my feet. There is nothing like having a very caring and thoughtful son-in-law. It's one of those things that makes a trip to the hospital feel a little better. While walking the halls my son-in-law met a gentlemen with both lungs down and introduced him to me. We made a fast friendship, and at this time, he introduced us to his girlfriend Katy. He had a rare lung disease. Adversity and suffering make for good friendships. Though neither of us knew it then, our doctors did not think either of us would leave the hospital alive. Both his lungs had collapsed. The affliction had caused his lung linings to be eaten away. The doctors came up with an idea to pour special glue down the tube that went into his collapsed lungs to go around his lungs and reseal them. We were both determined, however, to go home to our families for Thanksgiving. We made our rounds, shuffling down the corridors dragging our IV's and lung machines, looking more dead than alive, but we talked and walked just the same.

On Nov. 12th I had a bone scan and another chest x-ray. I never could understand why I had to have all these chest x-rays, but they were necessary to the doctors.

Nov. 13th was supposed to be a day of rest. Tell me, who's ever gone to a hospital and had any rest? They come in early to tell you to get ready for breakfast which arrives in another two hours. Then during the night they come in to take your temperature and blood pressure, waking you up. But the one I like best was when they came in and woke me up to tell me it's time for a sleeping pill.

On Nov. 14th the oncology staff gave me a major consultation. Dr. Butler was in charge and when he finished around noon the hospital staff was taking him out to lunch, as it was his last day. I believe I was his last patient. He was leaving the hospital to go out on his own. This is when my 60-day notice to live was given. They also asked me if I would become part of an experiment.

Being diagnosed with a terminal illness they could experiment with my body, using me like a guinea pig. All over the country 47 others also would participate in this experiment.

My first thought was would it help other people? When told that it would, I consented. I felt at least then my life would not be wasted if I could help other people with cancer. The experiment was to consist of very strong doses of chemotherapy, followed by surgery and then followed by radiation and chemotherapy for two years.

After getting the news of how short a time I had to live, that night laying in my bed, I had a long talk with my God. I said, "Lord, You'll have to go with me through this as this is a heavy load. I would certainly appreciate You giving me a miraculous healing, a real miracle, but, Lord, if that's not in Your plan I will take my healing anyway You give it to me, as long as You stay with me. But if it's my turn to die I'll see You in a couple of months." I decided to keep it to myself for a few days. Three days later, I told Mary, but asked her not to tell our children Ted and Tammy.

"We'll tell them after I get out of the hospital," I said. I felt the hospital setting was not a good place or time to tell them such news.

Mary did not take the news very well: not quite ready to give up her partner! We were to the point where we felt the two of us had become one. She would feel as though she was half a person. Driving home through a flood of tears, she was thinking of the good times and not wanting them to stop. She arrived home, got through the kitchen door and totally broke down. Mary didn't want to remove her coat or stay in the house feeling that she didn't belong there anymore. It's over.

Full of mixed emotions I slept very little. I was praying in the hospital and I think this made a difference. People die praying for God to heal them, including my friend Roland. People seem to think that the only way God heals them is through divine healing. They don't realize they are tying God's hands. Can God not use a physician? In the Old Testament he performed the first surgery on Adam. Another time of healing in the Bible was when Christ healed the blind man. He used spit mixed with clay and anointed the eyes. You can read this story in two places in the Bible. (Mark 8:23 & John 9:6) Wouldn't the spit be the same as an ointment applied by the divine hand of God? He healed in a lot of ways, and we fail to see that, and think the only way was divine intervention. I said, "Lord, I would like a divine healing, but if it's not Your will, I will go through treatment until You intervene. I don't care if my healing is from the doctor, from medicine, from radiation, from chemotherapy or through the surgeon's hands, they all can be Your means of healing." But I! I would like! divine intervention. I would like not to go through these things. So as I went along, before the next phase, I would always say, take another x-ray to make sure it's still there. I was hoping and praying that He intervened. But if He didn't, I was ready for the next step. I knew He could do it, and I wasn't about to tie His hands. I would accept it any way, shape, form or manner, and I kept looking for evidence of His faithfulness.

In my case He let me go through treatment until I had two more years of chemotherapy. At that point it's as if He said, "You proved you would go this way so I'm going to heal you at this point, so you won't need the two years more of chemo therapy."

## Chapter Six

# Looking to the Future

Having just been given two months to live I decided to start planning a trip to Florida one year in advance, so that I would have a long term goal to look forward to.

Nov. 15th, in the hospital. In the morning I went down for a chest scan and late that day a liver and spleen scan. Sometimes as you go through these tests, you think they're worse than the disease itself. You spend your time in the room waiting to go for the tests or someone to come to your room and tell you about the results of prior tests.

Nov. 16th. They decided to do a head cat scan. You lay flat on your back and they put these big clamps on your head so you can't move. Then they want to stick you in this tunnel and leave you in there for an hour. In all that time I looked and looked but I never did find any cats. Maybe you'll have better luck.

Nov. 17th. I must have failed the other cat scan so they did a whole body scan. This time strapped down like Frankenstein and back into the tunnel for over an hour because I hadn't found any cats the day before. Evidently they were giving me a second chance but I didn't find any then either. But what they found was a hot spot on my knee, which means I either had another cancer or arthritis. It would require surgery to know which one it was.

So what was Mary doing? She went bowling feeling very emotional. I wanted her to keep a normal life as much as possible. While there she did a lot of crying, as everyone was asking a lot of questions about me. She didn't bowl very well, but being around friends helped a lot. Her heart was at the hospital; just her body was at the bowling alley.

Nov. 18th. In preparation for the knee surgery that would be coming up on the 21st, I had some knee film taken. After that I had to go once again for a chest x-ray.

By this time Doctor Ron Cone, our dentist friend from Full Gospel, and many other friends and church members visited and prayed with me in the hospital.

Mary went to dinner at a Brockport diner, as Tammy and Bill were living in Brockport at the time. After supper Tammy and Mary had some personal time as Bill went home with Crystal. Although no appetite for it, Mary tried a dish of ice cream while discussing life's situation. Nothing worked and tears kept coming. She just wanted to hide. She could imagine what our daughter Tammy was feeling. They still had some comforting words for each other. Later she went to Tammy's and stayed there a few nights, as life was so lonesome without me at home.

Nov. 19th. Still in the hospital, I awoke, got up and found my clothes and got dressed. Since it was Sunday, I told the nurses I was taking the day off. I took Mary to the hospital cafeteria for lunch. All the nurses knew I was terminal and allowed me some freedom. While having lunch the conversation was mostly about how to handle the new circumstances that we were facing, knowing life would be different here on out. Then we went to an enclosed garden within the hospital, sitting among the pretty flowers and landscape we were no longer thinking about ourselves. We were absorbed in the beauty around us and in the fresh air. We even walked awhile outside the hospital. It was wonderful in the midst of a storm. It's great to know that your anchor holds.

Then my brother Harry and his wife Jean came to visit and presented me with my "feelings book" to keep track daily. It came in handy for writing this book. I wouldn't have had all the details and dates. Thank God for brothers.

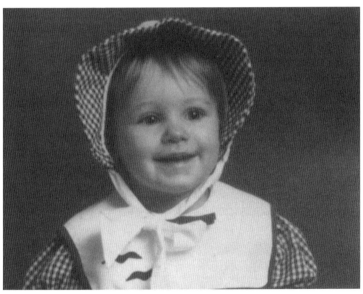

Our sweet inspiration, Crystal, who helped us through.

One thing I got to do was entertain a very special visitor almost every day. At 18 months, my granddaughter Crystal would normally be restricted from seeing anyone in the hospital. She came almost daily, however, to sit on the bed and play for hours. We talked, we took naps and ate together. She became such an inspiration that the staff allowed her to freely come and go. Every time I saw Crystal I thought about life and how precious it is. Here's new life coming in to take the place of this old body that may be going out. She was the greatest inspiration in this world and there is and always will be a special place in my heart for that little one. I didn't expect to see her attend kindergarten and now she's in Calvary Chapel Bible College and I'm still here. Hallelujah!

The nurses in my area were some of the nicest in the whole hospital. They knew I was terminal and going through a lot of tests at all hours. They would stop in all through the night and sit on the bed and talk. The "day nurses" let us get away with a lot. For example, Crystal spending time with me and going to the cafeteria.

Nov. 20th. Harry and Jean spent the evening before with Mary and left to go back to the Catskills. I got dressed and Mary and I went to the hospital cafeteria for something to eat. Knowing I'd be going for surgery the next day relaxed us a bit. It was a tough night sleep for me.

Nov. 21st. After a nice breakfast they did a BX Tibia. In the afternoon I went for the knee surgery. They opened up the kneecap and moved it out of the way so they could insert this large needle into the bone and extract bone marrow. The sample was sent out. It came back in two days and it was a good report. The hot spot was the result of a test that I had after I drank radioactive fluids. As they passed through the body they would create hot spots that were either cancer or arthritis.

Ironically had this hot spot been cancer I would not have qualified for this cancer experiment and treatment, because you could only have one localized spot.

Nov. 22nd. I am still in the hospital. Dr. Asbury stopped by for an oncology follow-up. This was my first meeting with him and he was taking over since Dr. Butler had left. I liked him from the beginning. He was very professional and very human. He seemed to have a heart for your hurt. While he was there, he scheduled an appointment with me for Dec. 5th. I was driving my doctors crazy because I wanted to go home for Thanksgiving. Even if they had to bring me back in I wanted that one day home with the family. Thanksgiving had always been a family tradition. I didn't want to miss this one because it might be my last. Around four o'clock the doctor came in and told me I could go home the next afternoon. Two days before Thanksgiving I gave my daughter, Tammy, money to go out and buy decorations.

On Wednesday, Nov. 23rd I left the hospital at noon to celebrate.

# Chapter Seven

# At Home - Day to Day

Nov. 24th, Thanksgiving Day. Because of the knee surgery I was given pain medication. Because of the pain, and being unable to bend my knee I had to take quite a bit of medication just to sit at the table with the family.  It sure was great to have everyone together. I was realizing again that it is the people in our lives that mean more to us than anything else. After a wonderful turkey dinner with all the dressing, I told Ted and Tammy and their spouses how bad the situation had become.

"With this type of cancer," I explained, "I probably have only two months left to live." My daughter, Tammy said, "I'm not ready to lose my Dad."

Oh my, I might not even see Christmas.  I also mourned the fact I would not see Crystal grow up.

Nov. 25th. I've been in a great deal of pain from the knee surgery and can't walk so it was pretty tough on Mary. Although I know she wanted to help in every way this is where she showed her love. She wouldn't have given up a moment of it. Because I was home and alive it meant so much to her. She came up with the idea to use our desk chair (on wheels) which made it easier for Mary to push me around the house.

Nov. 26th. Through all of this, with the pain in the foot and the thoughts in my mind, I don't sleep very well. Thank God for my family and friends who would stop by and help cheer me up. This day Crystal stopped by and she brought her parents with her, not bad for an

18-month-old child. I didn't like to see her coming down with the croup, making her sick. In the afternoon the house was a little quiet and Mary wanted to bathe me in the tub. It had been awhile since a tub bath (a sponge bath doesn't do the trick forever), so I was looking forward to this. It was quite an ordeal. As we look back, we can't remember how we accomplished it, but once we did it became a daily task.

Nov. 27th. The pain in the knee has gone down into the foot and I was having a great deal of problems with it. Sleep was bad before but now getting worse.

Nov. 28th. The foot pain was so bad I had to call the doctor. He prescribed pain medicine that I had from when I was released from the hospital to hold me over until the 2nd of December, as this was as soon as they could see me.

Nov. 29th. The pain became so bad I have an emergency appointment at 10:00 a.m. The pain medicine just wasn't strong enough.

Nov. 30th. They prescribed better medication, but with the cancer medication and the pain medication you're never quite with it. You seem to be in a fog most of the time. I was still not sleeping well.

Dec. 1st. I went to watch Mary bowl. It's amazing how many emotions are stirred by doing such a simple thing as going to watch somebody bowl. Of course everyone in the bowling alley knew the situation. They had a hundred questions. We answered what we could. It certainly was a great feeling to know that so many were concerned about me.

Dec. 2nd. Here's another one of those strange stories. Sometimes they just make you wonder what's going on. I went to Dr. Dickerson, my knee surgeon, and had x-rays taken. The nurse came back saying that she had to redo them, because they were lost. She had checked every conceivable place in the office but had no luck finding them. The nurse asked me if I was a warlock. She said that as long as she had been doing this she had never lost a single x-ray. Evidently she was proud of her record until I came into her life and ruined it. A second set was taken and they were O.K. The doctor said I could start weaning off the cane, but to be cautious for the next ten days and very careful for the next two months. No running or jumping. (The knee healed so well that in three months time it would be very difficult to find the scar.) After all this good news we went shopping to buy our Christmas presents for my brother Bob and his family up North. We left about 8:00 p.m. to go north and drop off the presents and pick up Chancy, Mary's Dad, for the winter. We stayed at my brother Bob's for the night.

Dec. 3rd. I woke up at my brother's house and had a nice breakfast, prepared by Sharon. We were all sitting at the table with our coffee discussing all these new events in my life. I found my brother and sister-in-law to be very concerned for me. Once again it's very important to have a supportive family. Right after lunch we took a nice ride from Adams to 1000 Island Park where we picked up Mary's Dad. Then we made the long trip back to Rochester.We got back around 10:30 p.m.

Sun., Dec. 4th. We managed to get up for church. Mary, Chancy and I went to Maranatha Fellowship in the old Greece Grange Hall. It was a very friendly and supportive group. The Pastor, Paul Colosi, had come to the hospital a few times to visit and pray with me.

## Chapter Eight

# Going through Chemo - Day to Day

Dec. 5th. This experimental program required very large doses of chemotherapy before the surgery to kill the outside of the cancer so that it can't give off those deadly seeds. The doses were so strong, there was no medicine strong enough to keep you from being sick. While taking chemo, they have to keep checking your blood count, because your body has to maintain a certain level. The first dose of chemotherapy consisted of: Doxorublein-Cytoxan and VP-16-213. I was given compazine for nausea. When we went in for the first dose we were frightened, but the nurses tried to help me relax. When they called my name to have me come in I sat next to a little table on which were five needles. Three of them were large enough for a horse, probably about six inches long (just the fluid collecting area); and probably an inch sticking out the other end. Right away I was thinking they couldn't be for me. I wondered how they would get a horse in there. Oh O.K. I guess I'm the horse. Thank goodness they put an I.V. in me and injected the needles through the I.V. The minute the chemicals started to flow I could taste it in my throat and it tasted like metal. They tried to help with hard candy on standby. After it was over I went home and felt miserable right through the night.

Dec. 6th. Sickness continued all day and into the night. I got up and started throwing up. I said to myself, "Chemotherapy is not going to be fun." It's terrible walking around with this queasy feeling. Maybe this would be a good time to explain why they used three different fluids for the chemo. They found with one kind the cancer would figure it out and become immune, so they went to two and the cancer managed to figure it out and become immune to both kinds. By using three, they found the cancer couldn't figure them out and couldn't become immune.

Dec. 7th. Time to go back for another dose of chemo even though I'm still sick. I got to the hospital and made it in time to run to the bathroom and throw up. Then they ran some tests and said they cannot alter the chemo schedule and that they would still have to give it to me. You could see the sympathy in their eyes as they told me this. They changed the medicine for my stomach from Compazine to Valium. That seemed to work much better. When I got home I exercised on a stationary bike a little, and I ate a lot. Knowing I'd be losing my hair the doctor gave me a prescription for a full hairpiece.

Dec. 8th. I'm feeling much better. Of course going so far down after the chemo any improvement feels great. I'm sure this may not be for everyone, but I found that I could eat and keep down chicken noodle soup. In the morning I would have breakfast cereal and then for lunch and supper, chicken noodle soup.

Dec. 9th. I went in this morning for chemo. I can't believe it but it was a little easier thanks to the Valium, chicken noodle soup and some exercise that seemed to help digest the soup.

Dec. 10th. My son and daughter-in-law stopped by with the idea that maybe walking would be even better exercise. So we all went over to Marketplace Mall and I got in some good exercise and we had lunch. I will try this more often. You have to experiment with these things as to what to eat and what to do, like exercise, because nobody has been in this position before.

Dec. 11th. I got up this morning and went to Maranatha for church. The post card club had a meeting and they were electing officers. I had been involved with the club for quite a while so I did not want to give it up. It helped to keep normal activities in my life. Anything that can help keep your mind active and from thinking about cancer.

Dec. 12th. A busy day. I had an early appointment at the hospital for lab work and Mary went to TOPS which stands for (Take Off Pounds Sensibly), as she had a small weight problem. After weigh-in and meeting they would go out for lunch. I got out of the hospital in time to join the girls for lunch. After that I had an appointment with Dr. Craver to set a date for lung surgery. That was set up for Jan. 27, 1984. Then on to an Agape dinner at Maranatha. It was very good.

Dec. 13th. A good day because Channel 21 came over to our house to do a story on Chancy and his decoys. It is amazing how much a film crew can interrupt your life with all their lights and equipment. They did a very good job on the subject. It was just a short subject on the human side of the news. After all this disruption Chancy wanted to take us out to supper. We said, "sounds good to us." He wasn't accustomed to doing this very often.

Dec. 14th. We started out with a list of gifts that people would like for Christmas and went shopping. We were in the right part of town to visit the fellows I worked with at Rochester Products. We stopped at a little eatery for a quick lunch so I could go in and see them. They were surprised. Everybody was throwing questions at me from all directions wanting to know how I was making out. So I took the time and described how miserable that first dose of chemo was but that I was feeling much better now and was back to sleeping fairly well. They all wanted me to come back for a visit, preferably after my two months was over. They wanted to see if I would make it.

Dec. 15th. Mary and Tammy are both on the same bowling team. They wanted me to come and watch since they were doing great in first place. After bowling Tammy and Crystal came home with us and stayed all night because we needed help. Tammy was our helper. We had Christmas cards to get out. She did a great job with all the cards because at this stage it was a little difficult to get in the Christmas spirit, with cancer on your mind.

Dec. 16th. We went grocery shopping and started to get in some of the items needed for Christmas dinner. That evening we had a neighborhood annual Christmas party at Judy's, just down the street from us. We had a real nice time. As always Chancy was invited since he was with us winters. Judy was a born-again Christian for real and she was always praying for the people in the neighborhood who had problems. Judy also held Bible studies in her home. What a neighbor she was. We miss her since we've moved.

Dec. 17th. This morning we got up and went to a Full Gospel Businessmen's breakfast. A lot of friends were there who all wanted to know how I was doing. I told them I was doing pretty good. They all got around me and said a lovely prayer. How great it feels when you're surrounded by prayer. Now let me tell you a little thing about prayer I've learned while going through this. There is a different feeling with different people. Some people do it mechanically, just to make you think they have a concern, but you can feel it's not sincere. Other people will pray for you and there is love in the room because it's direct from their heart for you! That's the way it was this particular morning.

Whew! After we went Christmas shopping. Then we went to Brockport Hospital to visit Roland's son. At this time Tammy and Bill were living in Brockport so we paid them a visit. We got two birds with one stone.

Dec. 18th. We started out to go to church at Maranatha, but it was canceled because they were sharing the Grange Hall and the Grange decided to have a pancake breakfast that morning. Their building so it was their choice. Since church was canceled we decided it was a good time to visit Roland's wife. I had been so busy and so sick I hadn't had a chance to sit down and talk with her. We had a nice long visit. We reminisced about the trips and good times we used to have. Then later that evening I started coming down with a cold.

Dec. 19th. I got up this morning with that cold getting worse but I had to go in for lab work. They're always doing lab work and x-rays on me. I swear they keep a closer eye on me than the guards do on the gold in Fort Knox. I had a lot of pain in my lung, no one knew what was causing it, and I went to see Dr. Craver. He said I had pleurisy, nothing to worry about. That was the first day of having a bad hair day, the first I noticed it was falling out. This cold was getting a little worse. Believe me, when you have lung cancer you don't want a cold in your lungs.

Dec. 20th. I had an appointment for a hairpiece. It had been ordered and was supposed to be ready this day, but it wasn't. My hair was falling out much faster. I took a bath and washed my hair and it clogged the drain, so much had fallen out. My cold is getting worse. This evening I took some Comtrex for the cold.

Dec. 21st. I got up this morning and saw that the pillowcase was just covered with hair. Mary has to wash all the bedding daily as my hair is now falling out by the handfuls. I was very surprised to find out what it means to lose your hair, even when you know it's going to happen. It's one thing to go into the barber shop to get a hair cut, it's another when it comes out by the roots. When someone says you'll lose your hair from all these treatments you just automatically think it's from your head. But they mean every hair on your body. When I say that I mean every hair on your body and it's hard to grasp. The only hair left on me was my eyebrows. I don't know why that is. The emotions you go through are surprising. You almost feel that someone is taking you apart bit by bit. This was something I wasn't expecting. If somebody had written this out like I am now doing I think it would have been easier for me to go through the hair loss.

Dec. 22nd. I got up and had breakfast. We were discussing if the cancer does take me we had better make sure our wills are in order, (not that I thought by doing so I was giving up). I had no sense of giving up but only a fool would not take care of his financial house at a time like this. I just wanted to get this out of the way and on with my life. So we saw the lawyer and took care of the paper work. Mary had a gynecologist appointment. She was given a pap smear and the results came back not good. Keith, a friend from Rochester Products, stopped by with a big beautiful fruit basket from the fellows at work. My cold is getting worse and because of it I didn't sleep all night.

Dec. 23rd. The cold is so bad I was in bed most of the day. My hair is still falling out but a lot slower because there is very little left. My prayer was, "Lord, please heal this cold". My immune system was extremely weakened because of all the treatments, that's why I had the cold.

Dec. 24th, Christmas Eve. This cold is getting totally out of hand so I told Mary to call Dr. Asbury. He said to come into Emergency. They ran a test to see if it was pneumonia. While laying there my old doctor came in, puffing on a cigar. Twelve years earlier he had told me to stop smoking so as sick as I was I had to have a little fun with him. I looked up and said, "It's too bad you never went to my doctor. He would have told you to quit smoking as it's bad for your lungs. You'd ought to get a better doctor than mine, preferably. The last time I visited his office I got the terrible news that I had terminal cancer. Besides, when I asked him earlier what my chances of living were he said he didn't know of anyone who's ever lived." I had to pay for that wonderful news. I never went back to his office. Back to the tests- it was Bronchitis. The doctor put me on Amoxicillin/Bristol 250 mg.

We were going to have Christmas at Tammy's. So we had to call her and tell her we had to change our plans and if we had any Christmas at all we'd have to have it at our house. Tammy, Bill and Crystal came here and brought everything and spent the night. I feel good with guests in the house.

Dec. 25th. It's here! It's Christmas Day, the day we celebrate the birth of Jesus Christ. He is the reason for the season. The Man walking through this with me. So I know it's going to be a good day. Our basement had been done over into living quarters and that's where we put a beautifully decorated tree. There is something about the smell of a live Christmas tree that says it's Christmas. At this time Crystal is the only young one in our lives. We all managed to get up before her. That's a miracle because little ones do get excited about the presents. When she came down those stairs and saw all those presents, her eyes lit up brighter than the lights on the tree. When we saw that little face, huge smiles came upon our faces that melted our hearts with joy and made all the planning worth while! As I watched this I forgot my cancer and my cold. What a feeling came over me as the aroma of the Christmas dinner came rolling to me. Tammy planned the dinner and prepared it, as Mary was too busy with me. It was excellent! When we sat down and were eating the delicious food we were having great fellowship. It was just a wonderful Christmas! *MERRY CHRISTMAS TO ALL AND TO ALL A GOOD NIGHT!*

Dec. 26th. I woke this morning and noticed right away that I felt better. I wasn't totally myself yet but headed in the right direction. I was still filled with a lot of pleasant thoughts of yesterday and how great it was. Our old neighbor, Ted Vick, dropped by for a visit and our next door neighbors called and wanted to know if we could come over for supper. Why, that's like asking a child if he wants some candy. Ginny is a good cook. No convincing there. My hair is about all gone and my body's about as smooth as a baby's. Well there's one advantage, I won't have to comb or shave for awhile.

Dec. 27th. On this day we are bound for the hospital. I have to have lab work, EKG, and then on to chest x-rays. Next I had to see Dr. Asbury. Chemo was set back a week because of the Bronchitis. My brother, Harry, came to stay a few days. I am doing pretty good with my weight. I was about 170 lbs. when I started with the cancer. I weigh 164 lbs. which is good.

Dec. 28th. We got up and had planned to take my brother to the big malls. He lives in the Catskills and it is a little unusual for him to see the large malls. He enjoyed them. He wanted to take us to lunch. Tammy and Bill stopped by on their way to have some family pictures taken and got a chance to talk with Harry. For a few days now I have been riding the stationary bike and today managed five miles on it.

Dec. 29th. Mary made Harry his favorite breakfast of french toast. It makes a nice aroma in the house. It was great and after some more coffee and conversation, Harry decided it was time to get on the road. That afternoon I got on the bike and rode another five miles.

Dec. 30th. We had to go out shopping to get all the goodies for New Year's Eve. We had quite a list and it took some time but it was great exercise. Then we took the car in and got it all greased and oiled ready for the New Year. Flo, Roland's wife, had called and asked us to come over for supper. She was a good cook and it was a wonderful supper. We talked and talked for hours. She was coming to our house with her friend the next night for New Year's Eve.

Dec. 31st. Spent the day getting ready for tonight. 1984 is just around the corner. Our guests started arriving at 4:00. Dinner was at about 5:30. Tammy, Bill, Crystal, Teddy, Ellyn, Flo, and Lee came. We all had a great time until 2:00 or 3:00. Ain't it funny how time slips away.

Jan. 1st, 1984. We went to Maranatha today for prayer and fellowship to start the New Year. Everybody said a prayer in hopes of killing the cancer.

Jan. 2nd. Today is a real laid back day. Tomorrow I start up again with the chemo. So while Mary did a few things around the house, I did a little reading.

Jan. 3rd. Got up this morning, knowing it's chemo time. I had a breakfast of just a bowl of cereal because I'm afraid of throwing it back up again. I had a 1:00 p.m. appointment and they lost my records and didn't get out of there until 5:30 p.m. It's strange they lost x-rays and then they lost my records. They are going to give me my chemo and keep looking. They gave me a shot of Valium as they found this works best on my stomach. I was to take a tablet every four hours. I had the shot at 4:30 p.m. and the chemo about 15 minutes later. I went home very queasy. I had my bowl of chicken noodle soup. I laid in my Lazy Boy chair but didn't fall asleep until 3:00 a.m. I awoke again at 7:30 a.m. and was quite sick by 8:00 a.m.

Jan. 4th. I got up and took a Valium and tried to have breakfast. It was not going well. I kept the Valium up every four hours but it wasn't enough. I went to bed at 11:00 p.m., I awoke every two hours all night long because I was feeling so badly.

Jan. 5th. After a fitful night I awoke about 8:30 a.m. Still not feeling well. I tried to eat something again, I hoped it would help that queasy feeling. I took some Valium about 9:00 a.m. because I had chemo again today. My appointment was for 3:00 p.m They gave me 4 mg. of Hexadrol and 2 mg. of Haldol to take every four hours. It was like taking nothing. I was sick. So I went back to Valium at 4:30 p.m.

Jan. 6th. I was sick all day and couldn't settle down. I was wound up. I took some Valium at 4:30 a.m. I finally got to sleep around 5:00 a.m. and managed to sleep until around 10:30 a.m. I was sleeping in the chair yet because of the way my stomach was, I couldn't lay down flat. In the evening I started to feel better. The chicken noodle soup was kicking in. I took Valium at 11:00 p.m., went to bed at 12:00 and never got up until 8:30 a.m. That was the best night's sleep in some time.

Jan. 7th. As the day rolled on I started getting that sickness again and I never knew whether I felt that way from the last dose I had or because of the next dose coming.

Jan. 8th. I managed to go to Maranatha but was not feeling well so I requested more prayer just to help me get through the chemo. After we got home Mary did all kinds of things to make me feel better. It was another tough night for sleep because I have tomorrow's chemo on my mind.

Jan. 9th. I got up in the morning with chemo on my mind, this is like good news/bad news. The bad news was I had to go in at 4:00 p.m. for chemo, but the good news was this was the last chemo treatment before surgery. They gave me Reglan Hexadrol. I took another dose of this at 8:30 p.m. I weighed 162 lbs., which seemed like a miracle to me, because of not eating very well. I went to bed about 10:30, still in the chair but didn't sleep well. I was up a lot.

# Chapter Nine

# After Chemo - Day to Day

Jan. 10th. I took Valium throughout the day and still eating my chicken noodle soup. In the evening I tried Reglan Hexandrol but the medicine did nothing so I went back to Valium. It snowed during the night; I went out in the morning and shoveled for a little over an hour. There is something about exercise that helps to make you feel better.

Jan. 11th. What a difference a day makes. I went out of the house for the first time in over a week. I had to see Dr. Craver. He has to update all my records and says the surgery is still on schedule. They have to make sure my body is up to speed and my blood count is up to surgery. For those to whom this might make a difference I have noticed that if I exercise and eat chicken noodle soup I feel better. I don't know why this is, I just know it is.

Jan. 12th. I got up feeling good. This is Mary's bowling day so I decided to go and watch. Again at the bowling alley I'm attacked with questions. But it sure makes me feel good that somebody cares. Then we proceeded to the mall where we walked. I didn't make it all the way but it's that exercise thing again. However much you can do is good for you. We went home and had a decent evening and I slept pretty well. I didn't have to take any Valium this day.

Jan. 13th. I felt good in the morning and then it hit me and my spirits dropped and I felt terrible. I said,

"This is the day on which Roland passed away three years ago." So my emotions and my memory kicked in to high gear and we shed a few tears. Mary had an appointment to get a perm and I went along to learn about my hairpiece. I wanted to know how to take care of it. That evening we had some friends drop by. A lot of love and conversation, but when it came time for bed I didn't sleep well. Probably too many thoughts of Roland passing on.

Jan. 14th. Now that I'm beginning to feel at least human at this point, I should explain to you that these doses of chemo were above and beyond what most people would get. They are the whole key to this experiment as they have to kill the outside of this cancer in order to be able to do this surgery. This is also the reason why I had chemo before the surgery. I only had two Valium today.

Jan. 15th. Went to church this morning and Chancy went with us. After church we stopped at a restaurant for lunch and I found out something good. While I've been going through chemo the taste of coffee has been terrible and I'm a big coffee drinker. This morning I thought I'd try a cup. Wonderful! That will make your day. So it was a pretty good day. I only took one Valium at 7:00 p.m.

Jan. 16th. This is one of Mary's TOPS days. After the lunch ritual with the girls we went north to see my brother Bob. It was cold here but nowhere near as bad as in Adams. That night the temperature went down to 25 degrees below zero and they had a lot of snow. But we had a lot of warm friendship to take those snowy blahs away. No medication.

Jan. 17th. We woke up in Adams and went to the

kitchen for one of Sharon's fabulous breakfasts. One of the old landmarks of Clayton was the McCormick Restaurant. It had a fire so Mary, Chancy, and I had to visit Clayton to see how much damage was done. It had major damage and even damaged a couple other downtown buildings. Then we went back to Bob's and my sister Shirley came by. So I thought it would be a great time if we all went out to supper. There is something about going out to supper and conversation. The conversation is always nicer and flows easier. Maybe it has something to do with the fact that nobody gets stuck with the dishes. Anyway, it works and a good time was had by all.

Jan. 18th. I got up to another Sharon breakfast. Bob and Sharon hate to see us go so we didn't get on the road until 2:00 p.m. to come back to Rochester. That evening we had a dinner invitation at the Eckart's, one of Chancy's close friends. The three of us went over and the conversation went on until 11:30 that night.

Jan. 19th. Another bowling day for Mary. Their team is still holding in top position and it sure helps Mary get her mind off the things that are going on around us. Mary has a 1:00 p.m. appointment with her gynecologist. The doctor, when he did the exam, found some fibroids. He went ahead and burned them off in the office. I think he thought this would solve Mary's problems. It helped, but not totally. It went well for Mary but very difficult for me emotionally. I didn't want us both to be down at the same time. Going through the things I had been through my emotions were running high to start with. Our daughter and husband, stopped by to check on Mary because they knew she had a doctor's appointment. I'm feeling pretty good and only had to take one Valium.

Jan. 20th. This one is a busy day. I went to Genesee Hospital for pre admission testing. They took six tubes of blood, a urine test, EKG, and then off for a chest x-ray. That evening we went to Maranatha for fellowship. It started at 8:00 p.m. We never left until 11:30 that evening. Tammy and Bill went as well, so did Chancy. Everybody had a wonderful time, which should be recognizable by the fact that we left so late.

Jan. 21st. I got out of bed at 8:00 a.m., then we had to hurry as there was a Full Gospel men's breakfast, and we just made it. The guest speaker was J. Morris Smith. People had told him about me and the cancer and he wanted to pray for me. Jergen was there. He was a minister that stayed by Roland until the end. He has been with me through mine too. We had a long talk. That evening my stomach was a little queasy. So I had Valium at 5:30 and 11:30.

Jan. 22nd. We did things a little differently. Went to Jergen's church, called The Well. This was not the first time we had been to his church. This day the whole family went, including Chancy. When the service was over, we all went out for breakfast. They all came back to our house and didn't leave until about 4:30 p.m. The whole family had a beautiful day together. Mary made lunch for everybody.

Jan. 23rd. Mary went to her TOPS meeting and I went over and met them for lunch. It is nice to get together with all the women. I would say that a man makes out very well when his wife belongs to TOPS because all these ladies are excellent cooks, that's how they wind up at TOPS. They put on dinners and we men get to attend and are well fed by these good cooks. Everyone has a great time.

Jan. 24th. This is one of those quiet days where we spend a lot of time praying and contemplating the day of surgery and praying that it will go well. I only had to take one Valium in the afternoon.

Jan. 25th. I got up this morning thinking two days away from surgery. Jergen, also knowing this, came by around 4:00 p.m. to pray for me and get all the information to schedule when he should be there for my surgery. He was the first to arrive at the hospital even before the family made it. This man has a heart for hurting people as big as the whole outdoors. Some friends had invited us over for supper. That was very good because it took our minds off surgery the next day. We got home about 10:30 p.m. and didn't settle down for bed until around 1:00 a.m.

## Chapter Ten

# Surgery

Jan. 26th. I got up this morning and started planning for the hospital. This is my pre-surgery day so I had to pack up all the necessities. They wanted me to check in by 2:00 p.m. I thought it would be nice to go out for lunch. Tammy, Crystal, and Mary went with me. So we stopped at a real nice place on our way. We had a friendly lunch then on for check-in. Later that evening, Teddy, Ellyn and Grampa came to the hospital to see me. They no more than left and Mr. Eckart stopped by. While he was going out the door two men from Full Gospel Businessmen came in. They had come to cheer me up. But it worked in reverse. When they walked out they were more blessed and happy than when they came in. Everybody was gone by 8:30 p.m. The doctor came in for a pre-surgical exam which consisted of a lot of questions concerning my health. One of those questions was, "Did you ever smoke?" I said, "Yes, but the Lord had taken the cigarettes away from me about ten years ago." That's quite a story in itself. He made no comment but continued on with his examination. When he finished, he said, "I'm a Christian too," and then he asked if he could pray for me? I said, "You certainly can! That's the only way I'm going to get through this." They gave me a couple of sleeping pills as they wanted me to have a good night sleep before the surgery.
This is the story I told the doctor of how the Lord took away the cigarettes.

I quit smoking in 1974. It's a story of God's love. Prior to this my daughter was after me all the time to quit. I told her that God would take care of it. When she was around eleven years of age she wanted her father to quit smoking. By the time she was twelve she had started hiding my cigarettes. She was fourteen when I handed her my last pack with the last cigarette in it and said, "If I ever need it, I'll come to you."

The heart of a little child will lead us for they have pure love. It was great to have one who was that concerned and so full of love for me. This is what happened: I went to a Full Gospel Businessmen's breakfast meeting in Syracuse. Even at this time if I had gone to a movie I'd have to get up and have a cigarette a couple of times during the hour and a half. There was an afternoon session but I had a cigarette before going in. I came out to go to supper and after supper I lit up a cigarette. It dawned on me that this was the first one I'd had since I went in, which was three or four hours prior. I went back in for the evening session. On my way in I picked up another pack of cigarettes to make sure I wouldn't run out. On my way home that evening around midnight I was having a cigarette when it dawned on me that this was the first since supper. The next day being Sunday I went to church and I don't recall smoking. Monday I went to work and at the end of the day I always had to empty my ashtray. I noticed there were only three cigarettes in it. At the end of the next day there were only two cigarettes in the ashtray. That's when I realized that the Lord had taken them away. I had tried to quit many times before but never could. One time I had quit for three weeks but I got so irritable and so nasty my wife said either start smoking or she's leaving.

But when God did it, it was so sweet and gentle. There was one cigarette left in the pack and I still had the full pack unopened. I gave it away and the last cigarette I gave to my daughter and I said, "I'll never need them again." Thank God for setting the captive free!

Jan. 27th. Here we are on the day of surgery. The family got up very early, around 5:00 a.m. and stopped on their way for breakfast. They were not used to being up this early and they wanted to be at the hospital by 6:00 a.m. That's why they fit in a quick breakfast. When they arrived at the hospital Jergen was already there. It was so great for the family to have Jergen with them while waiting. The family, basically Mary, was feeling dazed. Jergen took over. He was the one asking the right questions to the doctors and nurses and informing the family. Bill, my son-in-law, arrived just before I went down. I was upstairs just waiting to go to surgery and all the family came up with Jergen to give me last minute support. Unbeknownst to me a girl was supposed to come and take me down for surgery. Instead she took off and we never found out what happened to her. Because she was gone it became the job of a very nice young fellow who was a Christian. He walked through the door and he and Jergen recognized each other right away. Seems he went to Jergen's church occasionally. He and I were talking all the way down to the surgical floor. They have holding areas where you wait until they're ready to wheel you into surgery. He put me in there and then turned to leave. He said, "Is there anything I can do for you?" I said, "Yes, you can pray for me." He did very efficiently. He stood at the foot of my bed and I found out he was definitely not a closet type of Christian. His prayer just came rolling out of him in a very loud voice.

63

It caused all of those white uniforms to come to a halt. Some were just listening and some bowed their heads and joined in.

Before the operation I was told I would be in intensive care for three days and another two weeks in the hospital. I was out of intensive care in less than 24 hours and on the sixth day went home. While I was receiving the first shot to knock me out, laying on my stomach, I looked up at the doctor and said, "I've been looking all over for one of those stickers that says, Do not open until Dec. 25th." You have to give them a little humor or they'll take themselves too seriously.

The family, in the meantime, went back to the lobby for that long, long wait. Again, it was great to have Jergen to help cheer them up. Their wait lasted until 11:30 a.m. when the news came. The family and Jergen were called up to the surgical floor. Dr. Craver came into the waiting area and said all went well. The chemo had done its job. It killed the outside and the seeds, then the cancer was sent out to a lab where they found the inside was very much alive. They only had to remove about 10% of the lung and there were no complications. Prior to surgery they had thought they were going to have to take the whole lung because there were cancer roots in it. Just before surgery things seemed to have changed; they decided they would only have to take half of the lung. It's great when God is on your side for He was causing the roots to pull out of that lung. When they got in there they found no roots at all. That's why they only had to take 10%. WHAT A BLESSING! Now the waiting was over and the healing began. Our son, Teddy, after hearing everything went well said, "I could have hugged that doctor." At this time I was headed for ICU. I was in

64

ICU and Mr. Eckart and Mary walked in. They were my first guests. Mary left soon after seeing me with all those tubes and the oxygen mask. After hearing there were no complications it was an awful shock to see how I looked after surgery. Leaving the room Mary went to Jergen for support, crying on his shoulder. Teddy and Ellyn walked in to see their dad for a short time. Then it was time for Tammy and Bill. Tammy took one quick look at her father in ICU and went running for the door. Mary passed her coming out as she was coming back in. She was very upset to see her father in that condition with all those tubes (about nine of them) and an oxygen mask hooked up too. It also was a very depressing place anyway! Tammy showed her emotions more than any of us.

They need you to urinate after surgery. It's a bit of a job to get the waterworks running again, one of those things a plumber can't handle. They were unsuccessful so they asked me to get on my feet. I got up and they could not believe it. They kept me there for about three or four minutes. This was done about three hours after surgery. The most painful part was when they put me back down in bed. They had to make sure I didn't lay on any of the tubes. They left me lying there for a while longer and when the waterworks didn't flow they inserted a catheter. I had a catheter going into me, my lung was down, so I had a tube going into the lung. (I told you earlier how much fun that was.) Five wires for the EKG on my chest, an oxygen mask, an I.V. of sugar water and an I.V. of antibiotics. They had put special socks on my feet for blood circulation. Something was hooked up for blood pressure. There may have been more but I don't remember. Then my friend, the clown, came on the scene. The clown is a machine into which you exhale to help blow up your lungs. It has a gauge on it that has different colors as you get higher and higher and when you get to the very top his eyes light up. At this time I was a long way from making his eyes light up. They were giving me morphine for pain. In ICU it is almost impossible to get any sleep as there are people coming and going 24 hours a day. You would hear new emergency patients coming in. They'd be crying and screaming. So I'd lie still and pray for them. I prayed for myself. There were no windows, no clock that I could see and the unit was lit up all night long so I didn't have a clue as to what time it was. They kept working on me a lot of the time with the clown. All meals were liquid. Relatives were allowed only 10 minutes every hour only two at a time. The Leecy's came to visit the family in the ICU waiting room. They couldn't see me, not being relatives. But it gave the family support and someone to talk to during those 50 minute waits to go back in. Nobody wanted to leave the waiting room. So our son-in-law ran all the way to McDonald's to get everyone something to eat. Mary and Tammy left about 10:00 p.m. There wasn't much more they could do. They would have stayed the night but Mary was quite sick with a cold and didn't want to give it to me. She knew with the Lord on my side and all the great doctors, I was in good hands.

Jan. 28th. Here it is, Saturday. It's very hectic in here today. They came in to give me a liquid breakfast. Not much, believe me. I'm still playing with the clown about every half hour. Mary, Tammy, Bill, and Crystal came to visit. Everybody got in to see me except Crystal and she was very upset because they wouldn't let her see her Pa. Dr. Craver told us I would be in my room by afternoon. Both I.V.'s came out and I had a liquid lunch.

By 2:30 p.m. I was in my room. It was a miracle I only spent around 24 hours in ICU. When we talked of this earlier they thought it would be a three day stay. Another answered prayer. The children left around 3:00 p.m. and at 4:30 p.m. Teddy and Ellyn came by my room and stayed until 9:00 and, of course, Mary was there too. (Time for another little story.)

When I was in the hospital I had two friends, Leo and Chuck, who visited me. Shortly after diagnosis I can remember looking up at them and thinking of how healthy and young they looked for their ages. They were both going out with their wives after they left the hospital. I laid there thinking to myself how lucky they were because all I had to look forward to at that time was death. Let me tell you now you never want to be anybody but yourself. You never know what trouble lies ahead. I was looking at it from one point of view and my vision was blurred by that dreaded word - Cancer, and a short life expectancy. Although they didn't know it at the time, their life expectancies were shorter than mine. Believe me, I miss them both as they were great friends. But it sure taught me a lesson. Never be anybody but yourself. God made you the way you are and that's the way He wants you to be.

Jan. 29th. A quieter day. The main thing was for me to work on the clown every half hour. One time I managed to see those eyes light up. I was beginning to think he was broken. I'd get so close on occasions but just not close enough, until that one time. The whole family was there visiting when it happened and it made them very happy, because now they knew that my lung capacity was getting better.

Jan. 30th. This was also an easy day. They were just busy checking my vital signs. I was still working the clown, only now it was an hour or so between. I had all kinds of visitors-a lot of pastors I knew as well as friends and family. That evening after it all quieted down, I was lying in my hospital bed when I got a wonderful surprise. It's a good thing I was lying in my bed, because I never thought I would see this guy again. It was the same doctor that gave me my pre-surgical exam. He just stopped by to check up on me, and had a story to tell me. It was a real neat one. It seems the day of my surgery he was supposed to come in as an observer. Here God must have intervened again, because one of the doctors that was scheduled to be there as part of the surgical team didn't show up. Strange, huh? He was moved in to take his place. He was quite excited to tell me that he actually had his hands inside my body while praying for me. It's just too good to be true!

Jan. 31st. This turns out to be a great day. The doctors stopped by to tell me there was a possibility of my leaving the hospital on Feb. 1st. Great news! Tammy, Bill, and Crystal had made arrangements to go to Florida to see Bill's parents. They were to stay just over a week, so they had to leave the hospital and get ready for the trip. They had worried about leaving me, but I said, "I'm doing fine now. If you don't go because of me, I will feel very hurt, because I want you to go and have a good time." Teddy had to pick them up by 5:00 p.m. to take them to Buffalo Airport.

## Chapter Eleven

# After Surgery - Day to Day

Feb. 1st. This is the day we've been looking forward to- being discharged from the hospital. The surgery's over and all went well. They put me on Percocet and Valium five times a day trying to control the pain. It's great freedom to be out of the hospital. Now I can sleep without a nurse coming in and waking me up for a sleeping pill. I also get to eat real food. Another one of those blessings. I was supposed to be in the hospital, in ICU, for three days and then in my room for two weeks and here I was leaving the hospital in just six days! It's a blessing to be home with the family. Because of the pain I'm taking it real easy. I spend a lot of time in my chair; it's more comfortable.

Feb. 2nd. We get up because there's a knock on the door. I opened the door and to my surprise there stood my sister Shirley and brother Harry. They came in early wanting to find out how I was doing. They stayed all day and left in the early evening. My son and his wife stopped by around 7:00 p.m. Then my friend Keith from work stopped and everyone stayed until about 9:00 p.m. It turned out to be a very busy day. We went to bed early and slept well.

Feb. 3rd. I got up a little late and over breakfast we discussed the plans for the day. I decided to go to Long Ridge Mall and try to walk as it had been some time since we had done it. I walked from the car into the mall, from the entrance into the main aisle, but at the first chair I saw, I had to sit down. It took about a half hour to get built back up enough to make it back to the car. I guess I was pushing myself a little too soon. As soon as I got home I went down for a nap. When I got up later I went across the street to my neighbor; we have the same doctor. She had breast cancer and now it was going into her bones. We made a great pair sitting around telling war stories of our treatments. It was nice to have someone close by who could relate. She's gone now. God rest her soul.

Feb. 4th. Got up this morning and discussed yesterday's events. This mall has become a real challenge to me. I am determined to make it all the way around it. It's great exercise and I need it. So off we go to the mall and this time I walked about a quarter of it. The pain was beginning to build up so I reached for my pain pills and to my surprise I had none. I was two hours overdue. Here I will insert a little information I learned. When taking pain pills you should take them on the schedule prescribed. If you don't, the pain gets a stronger foothold and it'll take more medicine to bring it back down again. This day was a fine example of it, because I suffered a lot of pain.

Feb. 5th. Went to church this morning and then back to the mall. This time I have company, Teddy and Ellyn. Even when I don't make it all the way it's great exercise and I do have to build myself back up. Making it all the way is my goal. It gives me something to look forward to. I got about half way today and had to stop because of the pain.

Feb. 6th. It's that day again when Mary's TOPS Club has their meeting. Mary goes with our neighbor, Ginny, and leaves the car for me so I can join them for lunch. I just can't tell you enough how good it feels to have good friends around you. You learn to value them more and more. Don't misunderstand me, having a loving family around you is first and your loving friends are second. I didn't go to the mall today, I was still getting over yesterday.

Feb. 7th. Here we go back to my challenge. It's time again to attack the mall. We no more than get started and I had to take a pain pill. I quit walking but we had to go to Sears to pick up a PowerMate head for the cleaner. So I went out to the car and drove to Sears because we couldn't make the walk. But we got it accomplished.

Feb. 8th. Today we have a job to do that we've been looking forward to for some time. We've got to be at the Buffalo Airport to meet a plane. That plane has some special people on board. It's Tammy, Bill, and Crystal who are coming back from their Florida trip. They came in right on time and Tammy was not feeling well. Actually she was quite sick. On our way home we had to pull off the road a few times because of Tam's sickness. Then we're told about Crystal. It seemed she was sick most of the time in Florida. We were very glad to see them, but felt badly about all their problems. Somehow Bill stayed well and took care of his family. By now I was way down on my medication, only taking a couple pills a day. Feels great!

Feb. 9th. After breakfast Tammy and Crystal stopped by. Tammy had a doctor's appointment at 3:00 p.m. She wanted me to take her. Mary stayed home with Crystal. When we got to the doctors Tammy went in for her exam. They came out to get me so I could hear the baby's heartbeat, something I had never had the privilege of doing before in my life. It just put me on cloud nine. This baby turned out to be my second grandchild, a boy, and he was named Robert Shadrach Cook. Robert is my middle name and Shadrach is from the Bible. He turned out to be another delight to our hearts.

Feb. 10th. Really starting to get back into the swing of things. We went out for breakfast and then to the grocery store. Got the car washed then set off to the bank. We stopped at the gas station and filled the car. This afternoon I have an appointment with Dr. Craver. After his examination he had me sit down in his office to tell me this story. After they removed the cancer the whole thing was sent out for tests. Today was the day that the results had come back and he wanted me to understand everything. Not only were the seeds dead but the outside of the cancer was dead. If this had been the normal way of doing things instead of the experimental way, they would have considered that the cancer was dead and I would be all set. But what they found when they opened this cancer up was that the inside was very much alive. They had accomplished what they had hoped to do which was to kill the outside and the seeds. When they went to remove it, it wouldn't spread. If it hadn't been removed it would have restored itself and gone on to end my life. The doctor said I was healing very well. What a nice consultation! Another note: Even with surgery and the removal of a cancer, cancer has a tendency to want to return to the original sight.

Feb. 11th. Another big day in my life. This is the day I climb "Mt. Everest." It may not be that great a feat to some, but it was to me. Since I started trying to walk the mall, this is the first day I walked it completely. What a total feeling of triumph for me to accomplish it!

Feb. 12th. I got up and went to church. I couldn't wait to tell them the story of how their prayers were being answered. After church I had to see if I could make it completely around the mall again. I did! It still makes me feel like I came in first in a 10K marathon. After that big accomplishment Teddy and Ellyn had a pizza party for us. This was the first time that a full day had gone by with this much activity and I had to take "0" medication. What a great feeling!

Feb. 13th. Today it's Mary's turn. She has the appointment with the gynecologist. She's told she's in pretty good shape but it's time for a mammogram. No bad news. From there we went over to the mall for our routine walk. When I got home, snow had built up on the driveway, so now it was time for a little more exercise. I and that snow shovel danced up and down the driveway until the snow was gone.

Feb. 14th. Valentine's Day. I would not let my sweetheart do any work. She kind of got the day off. We ate out, went to Denny's for breakfast, walked the mall, making sure I hadn't lost my ability. Then we stopped at Friendly's for lunch. It was time for Mary's mammogram. Everything was O.K. Since it was Valentine's Day, it made our hearts joyful and gay. Then we found out that the love of our lives was coming to spend the night. It's Crystal. What more could you ask for on Valentine's Day, than to have your little sweetheart come and spend the night. Not everything can go perfectly. What a day to have this happen. I had a filling fall out so I had to go to the dentist. They made an emergency appointment for 5:45 p.m. They put in a temporary filling. Now it's time to go and have supper with my two sweethearts. We didn't get there until 7:30 p.m.  Chancy went with us. We went to Denny's. A wonderful way to end a wonderful day. We got home just in time to put Crystal to bed and I wound up having to take Percocet.

Feb. 15th. Crystal got us up early. I still have my two favorite Valentine's. It's such a joy to have her stay over. I am sure blessed I have a whole family full of Valentines! I was still on medication, just temporarily.

Feb. 16th. I got the opportunity again to go with Tammy to the doctor's. This time I got to see Robert Shadrach on the ultrasound. Another one of those wonderful things that people get to do these days. When our two were born there was no such thing. So it really seemed like a treat. It made you look forward to his birth that much more. It made me feel like I couldn't wait. From here on we'll only highlight the important days when something medical happened or of major importance.

## Chapter Twelve

# Back to Chemo and Radiation: Important Dates Only

Feb. 24th. I was off the medication. After walking the interior of the mall I started working on the outside of the mall. Today is the first I accomplished the complete inside and outside. I've come a long way from that day I barely made it in the door.

Feb. 27th. I had a dentist appointment to have three teeth filled in preparation for the radiation. Dr. Calnon was a student at Strong Hospital. He had alot of training on cancer patients. When I told him I was going to get whole brain radiation he made it a point to have me come in to take care of every little tiny cavity. The radiation would cause those little cavities to get much bigger. It is amazing how we wind up in the right place at the right time. There is probably no other dentist that would have thought about it.

Mar. 1st. I got up in the morning and had a bowl of good hot cereal because I had to go out and shovel the driveway for the third day in a row. Good exercise. Tammy, Crystal, Mary and I went over to Strong Hospital to see a seminar called "Winning over Cancer." They had some very intelligent doctors and cancer experts who gave very interesting speeches. I'm living with what they were talking about but most of what was said went right over my head. So I didn't get very much out of it except to know when I write a book I shouldn't use any fancy terms in hopes that everybody can understand.

Mar. 2nd. I got up this morning to a clean drive-way. We go to Strong for their tour of the Cancer Center. This was very interesting. I believe this was a new Cancer Center and everybody involved with it was very impressed, which made us very impressed. They had a great information packet. We even went into the labs where they were beginning to make some breakthroughs on curing cancer. That also was a very interesting tour, very thorough. I had an appointment with Dr. Craver. I told him how impressed I was with what I saw at Strong.

Mar. 7th. Today is a big day for a little girl. My sweet inspiration, Crystal, turned two. Last night we got a call from Joe, the other lung patient. He wanted to get in touch with me because he thought it would be good for us to keep in contact. He remembered we both had Dr. Craver, because of the circumstances the doctor gave him our phone number. He said he'd like to meet at the Holiday Inn in Seneca Falls. We set up a time and we met. This was the first time I'd seen him since the day before Thanksgiving when I left the hospital. Found out he left Thanksgiving Day. After three or four cups of coffee and a lot of catching up with the news we went to a very nice restaurant in Seneca Falls. We were still chatting like a couple of old ladies over our surgeries. This is the area where Joe lived, so he took us on a tour of Seneca Falls, Waterloo, and Geneva. After that we went back to the Holiday Inn. He didn't want us to get lost so he took us back to where we started. We had to go in for another cup of coffee and more discussion on how our lives were going. We both felt pretty great for a couple of guys who shouldn't even have made it out of the hospital. It certainly made it a wonderful day!

Mar. 8th. Today we have a doctor's appointment. They did a lot of blood work, sometimes you feel like you're dealing with Dracula. Then some days it's easier. On for x-rays then back to the doctor for blood pressure, weight, normal things. After he completed this, we sat down for a talk. One of the main things I got out of it was that I was doing fairly well. Then he talked about other cases. He told me over the last five years in Rochester alone there have been 120 cases of this type of lung cancer, of which less than ten have made it even for a few months. Not very good statistics. But I kept believing with God on my side I would get through this. By now I've outlived my two month projection and each day, God willing, I'll add another. You really try to make each day count.

Mar. 11th. I woke up to more snow but managed to make it to church. Had a post card meeting which had to be cancelled due to bad weather. Later that day Tammy and Bill stopped by to pick up Chancy. We asked them to take him home with them for a couple of weeks because tomorrow morning I would be back into the chemo. I knew I wouldn't be too good and I wouldn't want him watching me while I was sick.

Mar. 12th. First dose since surgery. Went to Genesee Hospital for chemotherapy. I had to urinate and it was red. Although they are trying to make the chemo easier for me, the dose is about half of what it was. I took Haldol - 2mg. and took Hexadrol - 4mg. at 11:15 a.m., 5:15 p.m. & 11:00 p.m.

Unable to do much, was very fatigued, but I did not get sick. Thank God!

Mar. 13th. I was totally unable to do anything and I spent most of the day in bed very fatigued. I was still not getting sick. I took Haldol - 2mg. and Hexadrol - 4mg. at 8:30 a.m. and took Valium at 4:30 a.m. & 3:00 p.m.

Mar. 14th. Another unpleasant day. The hospital is waiting for me again so I go for my chemo feeling a little better than I had the last couple days. Just in time to make me feel worse again. We're on a roller coaster ride.

Mar. 15th. Another day back in bed with no energy, no ambition, just like I had been taking knockout drops. This chemotherapy business is not much fun. I pray God will take it away!

Mar. 16.th I went to Pat's across the street for coffee at about 10:30. She'd already been through some of these treatments. I was hoping that she would come up with something that might help. At this time you need somebody who's been there. She gave me some information on what to expect but not many answers as to what would help. Basically, I found out that all you can do is bite the bullet and move on.

Mar. 17th. St Patrick's Day. Thirty years ago today, Mary and I met, one of the biggest blessings in my life. Went to a Full Gospel Men's Breakfast. Bill Blakely was the speaker, then off to the Islands to take Chancy home. It was a little early and we just needed the space because of the treatments. Crystal was with us. When we got there we had to shovel about a foot of snow to get the car in. While waiting for the house to warm up, we went down to Aunt Violet's, Chancy's sister's. Then to Adam's to spend the night. Sunday morning we were at Bob's and then back to Rochester.

Mar. 19th. Mary went with the TOPS girls, then she had an appointment with Dr. Gandell and he informed her that she would be going in for surgery on April 9th. I stayed home and cleaned house since Joe O'Connell was coming with his girl friend Katy. They arrived at about 4:30 p.m.; went to Rick's for dinner. Came home for coffee; Joe said he was deteriorating and we gave him a copy of the Old Carver print.

Mar. 20th. We went to the dentist for a final check-up as the radiation is close at hand. Then we went to Rochester Products to fill out paper work for disability. On the way home I had to stop at the mall because today I felt well enough to walk it.

Mar. 21st. We went to Genesee Hospital to see Dr. Asbury about the starting of radiation and to deliver forms for disability which he in turn sent to Dr. Sobel. We walked Long Ridge Mall. After supper went to the library for books on cancer.

Mar. 22nd. Went with Mary for an ultrasound then shopping, she needed a robe for her hospital visit which starts tomorrow.

Mar. 23rd. We went to Genesee for an appointment with Dr. Sobel in radiation. He gave me a short physical and then a brief talk on the effects of radiation. The possible side effects are fatigue, headaches, visual disturbance, nausea, fever, skin reaction, hair loss, and loss of taste. Then he informed me that there is an 80% chance of cancer cells in the brain but after we radiate them there will be a 95% chance that there isn't any left. With odds like this, how can you say no? Then we went to social security about disability. We had supper with Roland's wife and then Jergen stopped by. It's just great to have a minister like this who cares.

Mar. 26th. We went to the Cartwrights to celebrate TOPS anniversary. Then came home to get ready to go to the hospital. X-ray the brain to make sure the radiation machine was set properly for brain treatment. No treatment today, but I was put on drugs to keep brain from swelling. They used half tablets of Decadron and then Tagament for the stomach because of the Decadron. Took (4) 1/2 tablets of Decadron and then took 4 tablets of Tagament. Valium at 12:00 a.m.

Mar. 27th. We went to Genesee Hospital for the first radiation treatment. After that we stopped at AAA for the trip to Disney. Took (4) 1/2 tablets of Decadron, (4) tablets of Tagament. Valium at 2:45 a.m.

Mar. 28th. Back to Genesee Hospital for second treatment. Took (4) 1/2 tablets of Decadron, (4) 1/2 tablets of Tagament and Valium at 1:30 a.m.

Mar. 29th. Back to the hospital for third treatment. Took same medication again. Valium at 12:30 a.m.

Mar. 30th. Forth radiation treatment. Same medication. Valium at 11:30 p.m.

Mar. 31st. We went to Peterson's wedding reception at the Mapledale. Very nice day. Then went to Tammy and Bill's for supper. Enjoyed the evening. Then I began to suffer with excessive gas from the medication. Took (3) 1/2 tablets of Decadron and (3) 1/2 tablets of Tagament. Valium at 1:00 a.m. and lots of Digel.

April 1st. I didn't sleep well Saturday night so didn't feel well on Sunday didn't make church. Still heavily gassed. Sunday night took (4) 1/2 tablets of Decadron, and (4) 1/2 of Tagament. 11:30 p.m. Valium and lots of Digel. My head is getting red. Mary said I looked like I'd been to Florida.

April 2nd. I stayed home and Mary went to TOPS, then down for the fifth radiation treatment - halfway through. Had to come home and rest awhile. Am still bothered with gas. I'm on the same medication again. Valium at 12:30 a.m. and Digel.

April 3rd. I weighed 172 lbs. Saw Dr. Sobel about the gas. He said, it was probably caused by the Decadron. I had the sixth treatment of radiation. Then I had to visit with Mary's Dr. Gandell about surgery at noon. We were to notify him the next day on our decision. That night we went to a Full Gospel Businessmen's Meeting and they prayed for energy level and it went up. Same medication.

April 4th. Ralph and Ginny took us out for breakfast at Denny's then had to go to the hospital for the seventh treatment of radiation. Same medication.

April 5th. I watched Crystal while Tammy and Mary bowled. Went down to Genesee for eighth treatment. Ellyn went with us. Same medication.

April 6th. In the morning we went to social security, still working on the disability. We stopped in at Maranatha. Went to lunch at Perkins with the Shaws. Pat Shaw, our neighbor, also had to see the doctor. Then we all went to Genesee for radiation-my ninth treatment. Also had lab work, EKG, and x-rays. Went to see Dr. Asbury, then went out later and walked the mall. Took (3) 1/2 tablets of Decadron and 3 Tagament.

April 7th. Saturday night we went to Tammy's and talked about the house and feel we'll get it appraised. We also walked the mall. Same medication.

April 8th. We went to church at Maranatha. We went to Burger King for lunch and went to a post card meeting. I took (3) 1/2 tablets of Decadron and 3 Tagament.

April 9th. I weighed 164 lbs. As if a treatment of radiation wouldn't be enough for one day, I'm also going to get chemotherapy. My last radiation treatment. But the chemo is supposed to be going on for two more years. When they gave me the chemo, I got a shot of Haldol and a shot of Decadron. I took (1) 1/2 tablet of Decadron and 1 of Tagament, pretty much out of it. I'm not sleeping well and I'm up at least once an hour and take 2 Haldol tablets.

April 10th. OUT OF IT! (3) 1/2 tablets of Decadron and 3 Tagament

April 11th. I had chemo, out of it most of the day. Up at 5:30 a.m. Thursday. Had 1 Haldol tablet and (3) 1/2 tablet of Decadron and 3 Tagament and Valium about 11:30.

April 12th. In the morning I got up and then went outside and planted flowers. Came in to answer the phone at 10:15 and I had to lie down. I didn't get up for three hours. Then some of the neighbors stopped by for coffee. In the mail today we got a surprise box of candy from Chancy. Took (3) 1/2 tablets of Decadron and 3 Tagament.

April 13th. I took Valium - 12:30 a.m. & 9:45 p.m. Last chemo treatment until April 30th. After lunch went to Gates Library and met the Pastor from Full Gospel. We went for coffee and donuts at Donuts by the Dozen. Then we took him, his wife and daughter home. Then started (2) 1/2 tablets of Decadron, 2 Tagament, and Benadryl.

April 14th. We went to a Full Gospel Breakfast. I wasn't feeling well. I took (2) 1/2 tablets of Decadron, and 2 Tagament.

April 15th. We went to Sherlou's Hillside with Teddy, Ellyn and Ellyn's parents to celebrate Teddy and Ellyn's first anniversary. They went from there to stay at the Marriott in Buffalo. Same as their wedding night. We got home and the Leecy's stopped in. I took (2) 1/2 tablets of Decadron and 2 Tagament.

April 16th. The lawyer called and he's going to initiate a claim on the accident. Mail came, bringing income tax check so we could pay off Tammy and Bill. After the Chiropractor visit we came back and Tammy had supper ready. Same medication.

April 30th. I had lab work, x-rays, and another dose of chemo.

May 8th. This is where God begins to intervene for me. I went in for blood work and x-rays but the blood work showed that I can't take this dose of chemo. I've got to get built up more as I'd been going through a bad cold. They put me on medication for it. They scheduled chemo for May 14th.

May 14th. Had to go in for chemo. We didn't know this was the last treatment. Actually I had two years to go, but God said, "You proved you will take the healing any way I give it. You have well proven it by coming this far. I saw when you were sick. I saw you take your chemo. I watched the radiation and I made sure I made everything work for you. So the next two years of chemo are on Me. You don't need it. So it's over."

John 11:4 says, "This sickness is not unto death, but for the glory of God."

## Chapter Thirteen

# On With the Rest of My Life

May 15th. The first time I went to Cancer Action was a meeting called "I can Cope with Cancer." Later, they moved to a beautiful home on East Ave. It was one of those gorgeous old mansions. It had secret panels, one of which was on the stairway, and it opened up to the office for the home owners. There were two sisters that had lived there all of their lives but now they are in a nursing home. Occasionally they bring them back to this house where they would give tours and explain what it was like to live there. As time went on, we got very involved with Cancer Action. They did a film on us.

May 25th. I had an appointment with Dr. Asbury for lab work and x-rays. He said, "You can't take the chemo." He didn't know it but I'd been told that so all he was doing was confirming what God had already said.

May 29th. In the middle of all this suffering and pain here comes another great blessing. This is the day that our daughter gave birth to our second grandchild, Robert Shadrach Cook. I woke up this morning very sick and I wanted so badly to go to the hospital where our grandson was to be born. But instead my son had to take me to a different hospital. Crystal went with us. Mary and Ellyn went with Tammy and Bill met them there. I got right in to see the doctor and he gave me a couple of shots, some pills and a prescription. We left and went right over to the other hospital to see our new grandson just as he was being born.

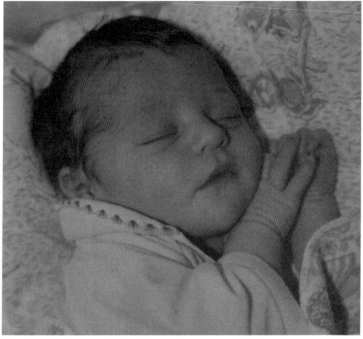

Our 1st grandson and I've always been proud of him. "Robert Shadrach"

May 30th. Appointment with Dr. Asbury for lab work and X-rays.

June 1st. Today it's Dr. Craver's turn to check my scar and my lungs. Since he's such a down home guy, we sat and talked a little while. He wanted to make sure I'm comfortable with it all and to know what's happening.

June 12th. Dr. Chey is a well-known stomach doctor, so I knew I had the best when I was admitted to Genesee Hospital because of stomach problems. I had memorized the menu because I was in so frequently, and told the nurse exactly what I wanted for supper that night. It was about 2:30 in the afternoon, and she said, "Let me see if I can get it for you." She went to the nurses' station and called the kitchen and told them exactly what I wanted. Lo and behold, when my supper arrived, it was just like I ordered.

June 14th. They did a spinal tap after my radiation treatments. Later I overheard this conversation I shouldn't have. Dr. Asbury, giving the spinal tap, and Dr. Sobel, who gave the radiation, were having a discussion. Dr. Asbury said he found gray matter in the spinal tap and he asked the radiation doctor if this had ever happened before. He said, "No".
Dr. Asbury said, "Have you ever had a patient who had a spinal tap shortly after whole brain radiation?" The answer again was "No." "Then you don't know anything about it either," but Dr. Asbury said, "there is gray matter in this spinal tap which must be brain cells." The whole brain radiation affected my memory. When it first started happening, I could be in my own backyard and not know how to get to the house or where I lived. Over time it got better but during this I couldn't go anywhere on my own. My wife had to be with me all the time. I couldn't remember names and couldn't remember what day it was. It's much better today, but I still need Mary while I'm getting around locally. Nowadays I can learn somebody's name, but it takes me a while to get it into my memory bank. It's a small price to pay.

July 6th. I had a follow up with Dr. Chey, the best stomach doctor in the world; they flew patients in to see him from all over the world. When I was in the hospital, the patient next to me was from Chicago. He had a severe stomach problem that the best doctors in Chicago tried to cure for three months and failed. Dr. Chey had him there for two weeks and sent him home healed.

July 10th. We started going to Make Today Count Meetings. In this group I became acquainted with a tennis pro. He got frustrated with his treatments and he went to New York City to go on a Micro Biotic diet. He came back to Rochester for a while and passed on.

Another gentleman I met while attending these meetings I'll refer to as the "orchid man." He used to bring orchids to the meetings and they were always beautiful. He even gave me a couple plants. He used to say, "I wish I had your faith." Now he's passed on.

There was another very nice lady with whom I had some interesting conversations. I enjoyed her but we didn't see her for a couple weeks. She called and asked if we'd all come over to her house for one meeting, which we did. She was on oxygen but she had enough tubing so she could go anywhere she wanted to in her apartment. It was good to see her up and around and looking good. But she passed on a few days later. I miss her.

July 13th. Today I had a double header. The first was Dr. Chey and the next was Dr. Sobel. After the appointment with Dr. Chey he told me to come back the 17th to find out how long it takes my stomach to digest food. He said to be there by 8:00 a.m. for breakfast. This sounded good to me. I'm thinking of ham and eggs and coffee. This was definitely different. Instead they gave me what they call a barium burger and then some of their delicious milk shake. It took me an hour and a half to eat this burger with the shake. After a certain number of bites and drinks they put me up against a machine to take an x-ray to see how the food was being digested. Probably if the food was real, they would get a real answer. This test went on for six hours and was only supposed to be an hour for the food to be digested. After all those hours, it hadn't started yet, so the doctor kicked me out. Later, I had a follow up with Dr. Sobel.

July 25th. I had an appointment with Dr. Asbury. First I went to the lab and they took six tubes of blood. Somebody walked in and said they needed four tubes of blood for a class they were teaching and they needed a volunteer. I said as long as you're already into my well of blood you might just as well drain off a couple more buckets. Then on to get x-rays. By now my stack of x-rays is so heavy that they have to give me a cart to wheel them back to my doctor.

Aug. 8th. Today's my 49th birthday and I'm hoping to see the 50th. I've invited the family over. Mary made a cake and a wonderful time was had by all. I really have something to celebrate, because I wasn't supposed to live this long.

Aug. 27th. Today is my daughter's birthday. Age unknown (she told me to say that). This evening we have a picnic with Cancer Action. Mary, my mother, and I are all going. Even though my mother has deteriorated a little more, she appeared to have had a great time.

Sept. 1st. We made it to our 28th wedding anniversary. The 28th does not stand out for most people, kind of inconspicuous. I'm not supposed to be here and if I wasn't here, my wife would have a big hole in her heart thinking of what could have been. Instead of that we had each other. We still had friends and family, all in life that is worthwhile; something to celebrate. We got a few friends together along with the family and went out and had a good time.

Sept. 3rd. I am finally well enough so Mary can have her surgery which was postponed a year ago because of my condition. It will take place tomorrow. The whole family was there, and it was supper time, so we went into the cafeteria to eat. Tammy, our daughter, got food poisoning from a tuna fish sandwich. That same night she was in emergency while her mother was on another floor after surgery.

Right after Mary's surgery, she had a good laugh while hurting. Before going into the hospital she had some sour milk, put in the back of the refrigerator for making cookies. Bill, our son-in-law, happened to be there one day and wanted a glass of milk, and got the milk out, and drank it all. By this time it was three weeks old, but he said it was good. Then when Mary returned home from surgery, Bill wanted to be of help, so he decided to do the laundry. One problem-the dryer wasn't working. So he strung rope outdoors and in, just full of clothes. What a great son-in-law, with such a caring and loving heart!

Sept. 5th. The doctors still keep me busy with appointments. Today it's Dr. Asbury and before my appointment I have lab work and x-rays. (Oct. 14, 1984 marks our first anniversary since the cancer was found. It's a great feeling to still be around.)

Nov. 1st. We went through the same routine as Sept. 5. After that, Dr. Asbury and I went into his office and we spoke about me going back to work. But at this time, he did not know if it would be a good idea.

Nov. 14th. It's time to go to see the radiation doctor.

Dr. Sobel was very different for a doctor. He wouldn't charge for the visit. He told his secretaries never to charge me. It was his privilege to see me because I was the only local person put in this program. He had high hopes that I would survive. I had a bad week this week because of the treatments, still suffering the effects of the chemo. It just seems to come and go. Now with all the troubles behind us it's on to better things.

# Chapter Fourteen

# Our Life After Treatments

On Nov. 18th. we went to St. Louis, Mo. to visit our friends, Ted and Paula Vick. Her Mom went with us. Paula's Mom was famous for her apple pies and she had made two fresh ones for her son-in-law, Ted. We were traveling by car and stopped somewhere in Illinois at a very nice restaurant. After we ate, the waitress asked if we wanted dessert. I said to her, "We have the best apple pie in the world in the car." She said their baker would like a piece of that pie.I brought it in, and told him to take only one piece. When she returned it, it was half gone. It seems the chef started bragging how good it was, so everyone had to sample it. On Nov. 19th. we just rested up from our trip. Nov. 20th. was Ted and Paula's anniversary. Over the next few days we took in the sights of St. Louis. The 24th took in the Fox Theater in the morning, went back on the River Boat for dinner and show. The waitresses and waiters were the ones that put on the show, it was great. Also went to the Old Railroad Union Station which had been restored with a lot of little shops and restaurants throughout. It was a very impressive sight to see one of these old railroad stations restored instead of bull-dozed. And of course when you're in St. Louis, you have to visit the Arch. It has an elevator that will take you to the top where you can view the Mississippi River or overlook the city of St. Louis. These are the highlights of those events. A very impressive sight was the completely restored Fox Theater. Years ago, it belonged to the Fox film makers. It was very elaborate. Our tour took a few hours. A millionaire purchased it and gave it to his wife to restore. Upon her first visit only one light bulb worked. When the work was completed, she had replaced over 10,000 light bulbs. Today it is used for all the big celebrities that come to the city. St. Louis was a great place to visit.

Now it's that time to take the Florida trip that I had planned for one year in advance, when first diagnosed with cancer. This trip consisted of Mary and I, my mom, my daughter, and granddaughter. We got up around 4:00 a.m. on Dec. 8th, 1984 to be at the Amtrak train station in Rochester. We arrived at Grand Central Station and had to take a shuttle over to Penn Station, carrying luggage for five people and trying to keep track of mom. While in Penn Station we had to get to the second level by escalator. Mom was in a wheelchair and wouldn't co-operate going on the escalator. A wonderful Red Cap saw the situation and offered help. He told us how to get around and on the train. He started talking to mom and had her settled down in no time. While she was turned in her wheelchair to visit with him, paying so close attention, she wasn't aware of what was happening. When we arrived at the train he had her still talking. We checked into Polynesian Village Hotel at Disney World and took the rest of the day orienting ourselves.

The next morning we went to breakfast in the hotel. On the menu was something new to us and we had to give it a try. It was french toast stuffed with bananas. Excellent choice! After breakfast, I bought a three day passport for two people. No way to get mom there in a wheelchair. One day my daughter and I chose to visit

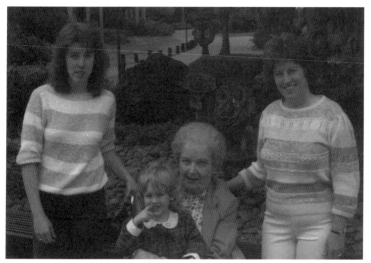

Tammy, Crystal, Nana and Mary in Florida. Ted's first one year in advance planning.

Epcot. Visited a lot of buildings and had a great day. The next day Mary, Crystal and I went to the Magic Kingdom. What a wonderful opportunity to be able to see the characters again through a two year old's eyes. Can it get any better than this? One day we got mom out on the tram rail and rode all through the kingdom so she could see it from her wheelchair. She was quite surprised going through a hotel on the tram rail.

The next day, Dec. 14th, had breakfast with the characters, Mom's face lit up about equal to Crystal's, like they were almost the same age. At this particular time Crystal liked to see the characters, but was afraid of them. I went over and talked to Minnie Mouse and explained the situation. They can't talk but they can listen; she attempted to approach Crystal and she started to cry. But before we left she had Crystal in her arms. Another wonderful sight to see, she never feared another character

93

from then on. On the 15th we took a trip to Cypress Gardens on a beautiful sunny day. Mom loved flowers and gardens so she was in her glory. At this time communication wasn't easy for her but all she had to do was look at all the beauty and it reflected back on her face. The whole trip was worth this one day. She had some good times, but this was probably her best. She even took their boat ride. Everybody went out of his or her way to help. We didn't want the day to end but with all days, it did, and we moved on. Now it's the 16th and time to leave, and as we look back on our trip, we are all commenting on the beautiful, beautiful Christmas decorations that were up all through Disney World. They were superb! Then to look forward to cold weather and snow back home. Everything worked as planned, and a great time was had by all. After fulfilling my long term commitment, it was time to plan another one. Being 49 at this time, I decided to plan a 50's birthday bash.

**In between our trips:**
May 22, 1985. I spoke at Teen Challenge. About a week prior to this I brought some more items into them and they asked me if I would preach to the boys at their morning worship. I accepted their invitation figuring I had a week to come up with my sermon. I started praying and asking God what to teach and nothing came the first day or the next. I started to get a little nervous. Nothing the third or the fourth days. Well, that's all right, I still have a couple days. Nothing happened. The day arrived and I got up with no topic and no notes. I'd have to totally rely on what God wants to do, fully expecting something to happen before the last minute. It didn't. They sang a few songs then turned it over to their guest

speaker, which was me. I remember standing up. I came this morning not to preach out of the Bible but to teach on faith. I didn't remember another thing until I ran out of words and turned it back over to them. The man in charge of Teen Challenge said my timing was perfect. We only had enough time for one song before we closed. What an awesome God to give me all the right words in His perfect timing. The boys wanted me to come back; they all enjoyed it so much. Of course they would; I wasn't speaking, the Holy Ghost was.

After walking out of Teen Challenge Mary remembered her Gramma saying that I would someday be a preacher. She saw me preaching dressed in a black suit. When I looked down I realized I had that black suit on. Mary's grandmother had truly received that prophecy 25 years in advance because at the time I was as deep in sin as anybody could be. Mary had just laughed when I was told I was going to be a preacher.

Even though my mom had Alzheimers and wasn't too sharp she still loved to go to the 1000 Islands area. She was born in Clayton, N.Y. in the same house where my grandmother, great grandmother and great-great grandmother lived. The area was home to her and she loved to watch the big steamers go up and down the river. We would make it a point to take her there once or twice a year for a few days at a time. She loved sitting on the balcony with a child-like enthusiasm when those big ships came thru. One of those times we took her was, June 6, 1985, to the 1000 Island Club. While there I was off taking pictures of Boldt's front farm property. I also took pictures of Boldt's polo pony barn where he used to keep his prized ponies. This building was in very bad shape. One picture was of a window with a board hanging down with one nail still holding and I called that picture "Soon to Fall." I felt like that board represented me because I was still going through treatment and the doctors were not yet confident I was going to make it. So I thought, which would fall first, that board or me? Shortly after taking the picture the whole building was leveled to make room for condos. It's gone but I'm still here. I also showed this to Dr. Asbury and Dr. Boros and they were very excited and wanted copies of it.

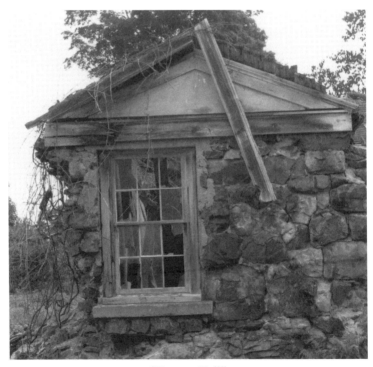

"Soon to Fall"
Taken June 8, 1985

# Chapter Fifteen

# My 50's Party

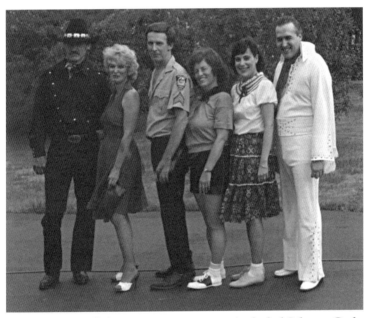

The "celebrities" that came to our party included Johnny Cash, Marilyn Monroe and Elvis.

My 50th birthday party in 1985 required a great deal of planning throughout the year. After the Florida trip we started because I wasn't suppose to make it to 50. I wanted to do it up right so everything in detail was oriented around the 50's style. In order to have enough seating we purchased cinder blocks and planks. One plank on blocks and one on the wall for support. We painted the garage pink and black. This included even the basement decorated with old car ads and pink and black balloons and streamers. We had hub caps nailed to the walls. (Also poster board up to my 50 years displayed memorabilia. The D.J. in a corner so he could display records on the wall.) We wanted everyone to dress like the 50's. The gifts were also 50's oriented, we even had trivia quiz of the era. The story of the day went like this; it began at 8:00 a.m. and went until 12:30 a.m. Over 100 people attended, some coming and going throughout the day. It starts out with a fun story. The disc jockey was there the night before setting it all up. He was ready to go at 8:00 a.m. the next day. He turned it on and cranked it up. Unbeknown to us at the time, our neighbor across the street woke up to the music thinking it was their clock radio. He tried three times to turn it off. In sheer desperation he finally pulled the plug but the music continued. They finally realized it was party time. The people who were there, were there for breakfast. Every half hour the D.J. had a trivia quiz and they would get up to three 50 cent pieces depending on the difficulty of the question asked going on throughout the day. There was also a pinball machine called Space Odyssey in the basement. People enjoyed that. In the evening there was a pinball contest and our son won. We had hots, hamburgers on the grill, and speaking of the grill, a neighbor and myself built one special for this party.

It was wonderful to see our children dressed in 50's style and participating as if they had lived as teenagers of this era. Of course this is the first 50's party, as later they had a second chance when they were at the Blast from the Past 50's party for Cancer Action. Our daughter was runner up for best dressed where she looked like Marilyn Monroe.

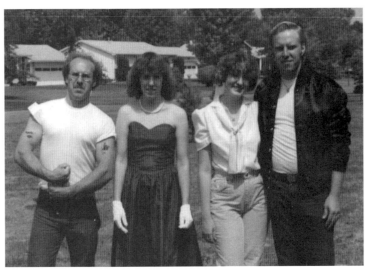

The nicest bunch of kids anyone could have.

Our very close friends Ted and Paula had moved to St. Louis and had stated that they were unable to make it because of something to do with Ted's job. They promised to do their best to get it changed so they could be here. At the last moment they called from St. Louis saying they couldn't make it. Shortly after noon the door bell rang and we looked and there was a large gift on the door step done up in black with pink bows. With great anticipation we went out to open it up. What a surprise, out popped Elvis (Ted) with his guitar. He came dressed like this on the plane. It's great to have friends that still love you when they move away.

After lunch the Holly Follies were there for entertainment. They were a dancing group, from 60 - 80 years old, who continually changed costumes for particular dances. None showed their age and were a big hit. We had a contest for the best dressed 50's outfit. The winner was Ted Vick and runner up was Joe O'Connell. The hula hoop contest was won by Katie, Joe's girlfriend. Of course dancing went on all day and really picked up at night.

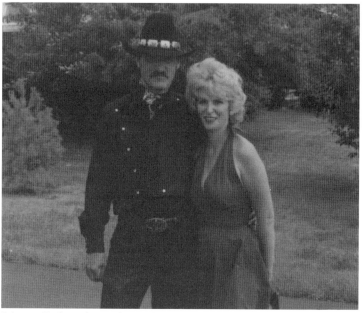

Johnny Cash with Marilyn. Johnny is the Joe I first met in the hospital.

We had a couple who heard about this party through a car club newsletter. Instead of going to the car show they decided to take in the party. They had more fun than any of the car shows or any other place they'd been with his car. They arrived in an old 1953 Chevy, all redone; a beautiful car. It looked nice in our driveway for our party. They were both dressed 50's style.

The people from the Donut Shop returned in the

afternoon to enjoy the party and when they came back they had an old 50's Dodge. They stayed with us until early evening. They couldn't believe the fun they had. Later in the afternoon Channel 13 showed up. They heard about this party where a man had been given two months to live yet planned his 50th birthday party. They thought it would be a good story for that evening's news. In the background of this report you could hear the 50's music playing as they interviewed me.

After this I opened an array of gifts. Some of the guests did an excellent job of staying with the 50's theme. One used fifty 50 cent pieces to spell out the number fifty. My neighbors got together and bought a five foot blue spruce tree and tied fifty $1.00 bills on the branches. Another used fifty- cent pieces to spell T.C.

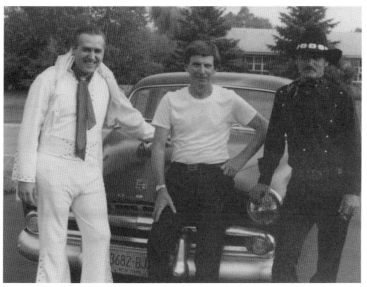

Elvis, Ted and Johnny Cash looking like the 50's.

This party was a big affair. Not very often do they last all day. We had breakfast, lunch and dinner, all of which went off well. As always, you save the best for last. We had so much going on this day we never got around to the birthday cake until 8:00 p.m. It was a big beautiful cake decorated in 50's style by Gruttardauria's Bakery. We all gathered in the basement to sing Happy Birthday and enjoy cake, coffee and great fellowship. Well worth all the planning! It made me cry. I don't know whether I was crying because the party was coming to an end or if my emotions from the whole day with all the great friends and wonderful gifts were ruling. Either way they were tears of joy. I just can't say enough of how wonderful and smoothly it all came out. Then everyone went back to the garage to finish dancing until after midnight.

## Chapter Sixteen

# Fun Times

Mary and I were on our way to Florida in the spring of '86. We were somewhere in N. Carolina and the weather was getting warmer. Mary said that she didn't like the hairpiece because it wasn't natural looking. She waited until we were in a warmer climate because the hairpiece helped hold the heat in. Supposedly 75% of body heat escapes through the top of the head. This brings up a point I don't talk about. Before I got the cancer, Mary used to call me her Armstrong heater, nowadays she's the Armstrong heater, as somewhere along the line treatments affected my body heat. In the winter time, if I go out on a cold day, you can put your hand on my body and feel the cold through the clothing. Just a small price to pay. I didn't want to give the hairpiece up, but I didn't want my wife to feel badly, so I switched to a hat. The first one had originally belonged to my Grandfather and was probably 40 years old at the time. I applied pins from different Christian organizations, my son's Air Force pin, and initial stick pin from my mom. It wound up to be about 35 pins in all. Needless to say with its age and all that weight it only lasted about 3 years. A hat for me to find was very difficult, because like my Grandfather, had a very large head. In the old days, if the back of your head was large, they called it the bump of knowledge. I know this was very true for my Grandfather worked at the NY AirBrake Co. and was credited with quite a few inventions. One was the hydraulics for landing gears and wheels on planes. Our size was $7\,^{7}/_{8}$ in a normal hat, but if they were special made a $7\,^{5}/_{8}$ oval would do. Now I should insert a note that goes back to the beginning. The original reason for the hairpiece was the way people look at you when your hair is gone. It makes you feel bad. It hurts to see the look in their eye, so in order to keep a more upbeat thought about yourself a hairpiece was best or a hat. Now the hair has come back in around the sides of my head but not on top. With no hair the heat loss is bad. So the hat contributes to maintaining heat throughout the body. A little story to go along with this: There was a lady once at Cancer Action who got very upset over the fact that I wore a hat and since I didn't want to offend anybody I took it off. It was summer which helped. By that fall that lady came up to me and asked, "Where is the hat?" She thought I should be wearing it. What a turn around. I put it back on and have been wearing one since.

One more hat story. I went to a Catholic wedding once and I was sitting in a pew before the festivities began when a man dressed like a priest came down. When he saw me he told me to get out. I said, "What's the matter?" He said, "You can't sit in this church with a hat on." He never asked me to remove it, just told me to get out. That's exactly what I did. I said to myself, "That man has no idea what I've been through and why I needed to wear a hat." Not that it would have done me much good to explain. Some people don't want to know the facts, they just want to condemn. As you go through life try not to offend someone without knowing the facts.

During all this my general practitioner retired. I needed to get a new one so I asked Dr. Asbury, Dr. Sobel, and Dr. Craver whom they would go to if they needed a doctor to see. All three gave me the same answer. They said, "Go to Dr. Schneider." So on Jan 2, 1986 Dr. Schneider became our family physician. Now our children and their families go to him also. He's a wonderful man.

Two and a half years later we took another trip to Florida for a month just to renew us. We stayed at the UAW Village in Satsuma, Florida. Rode bikes almost daily to build up stamina and strength. Some days got up and went to Daytona and walked the beach. While we were there, we took side trips to Venice, St. Augustine, Naples, and Sanibel Island.

Then in the fall, while Mary was bowling, we noticed a 1957 Cadillac for sale on Coldwater Road. After seeing it a few times, we thought it might make a good project for me to keep my mind off the cancer. It became a very elusive car. First we'd see it and then we didn't, and with my poor memory, I could never remember where I saw it. We finally purchased it in Dec. 1986. That is the same car that you'll read about in the story of the United Way film. It required a lot more work than what was first thought; but made up for it, in the fun we had with it.

In the fall of 1986 we won a trip to Jamaica, that we took May 1, 1987. Came back to Miami, Florida, May 9, then spent a week in Florida. Here are some of the highlights of the trip. After flying into Miami, I took sick at the airport, these things you expect to happen because of the cancer treatments. I was in the men's room until about five minutes before boarding for Jamaica and when I came out, Mary looked at me and said, "We'll cancel out, you're too sick to go on". I said, "I don't care if I

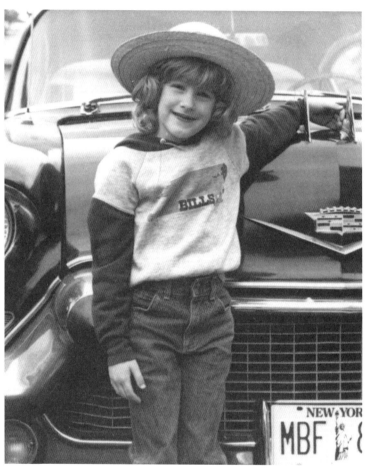

Dream Girl on the Dream Machine. Our sweet inspiration.

throw up all the way to Jamaica, I'm going now." Somehow I boarded the plane and arrived in Jamaica and after a day or so started to feel good again.

The resort we went to said they had a private island for a nudist camp. One day I had my camera out, looking for some interesting pictures and I stumbled on a beach area next to where we stayed and this was supposed to be the secret place. An awful lot of flesh showing, and no, we didn't take any pictures. We respected their privacy.

Another interesting event while we were there. They have a talent night and that's where they ask the guests to participate in a skit or whatever they can do. When they approached us we told them we could help with lights or behind the scenes. But they kept persisting we do something else. So being in Jamaica we got this idea if we said we'd sing, that they wouldn't have the right music. So they asked what song we'd sing, and we told them "One Day at a Time." Then we told them we didn't know the words, they would have to provide us with a copy and would you believe, they did, so we were committed. That night we're the last act, and we go out to sing; we've never done anything like this before. We started singing, started hearing the crowd yelling and stomping their feet. Mary tried to run off thinking they're mad or upset. But I hung on to her and said, "We're going to finish." Looking down at our words and the lights on us, we couldn't see the crowd. Mary was determined they were trying to run us off the stage. When it was over, the people gave us a standing ovation. The pounding we heard was for good and we thought it was for bad. They wanted to hear another song, but only had words for the one song. So we couldn't sing anymore.

The next day we were the talk of the resort and left for Daytona, where we spent a week before departing back to Rochester on May 16. We spent that week with my friend Joe, the fellow I had met with the lung disease. We had a great time. Everyday keeping busy.

Fun in the sun.

I don't want to bore you with a lot of trips to the doctors and a lot of tests, but they do still go on. I do have one I want to bring up. It was in March of 1986 while Mary was working at the Post Office and I was babysitting both of Tammy's children. Mary had left for work and I just started to get around. My feet hit the floor, the room began to spin and I ran to the bathroom, throwing up. I fell down to my knees, and couldn't get back up. Every time I raised up, I would get so dizzy I couldn't see. I dragged myself to the phone and called the Post Office and told them I was very sick with two children and needed Mary home right away. They informed Mary and she left immediately. She placed a call to the doctor and he said as soon as we could, see him. In the meantime, I had crawled back into the bedroom, and managed to get back in bed. If I even attempted to raise my head, the room started to spin, I laid like that for three days. Then it left.

I went in to see the doctor and then they scheduled an MRI. The results found a problem in the control nerve in the back of my head. This will be a great time to insert this information. I would have problems with this or that and I'd say, "Doc, how come this is happening or how come that is happening?" and they would look at me and say, "We don't know, we never had anybody live this long, so it's not up to us to be able to tell you, it's up to you to tell us." Kind of felt like a reversal of roles. It seems funny when it's up to you to tell the doctor instead of him having the privilege to tell you.

A little side benefit from all this cancer is that it caused my younger brother, Bob, to quit smoking. That was a great blessing to me to see that something good happened.

In the spring of 1988 we put our house on the market, the reason being, cancer was popping up all around us. The man we bought the house from was dying of cancer, then across the road, next to them, being on a corner, the other side, the couple and next door to them. Then skip a house and another case. Lots more up the road. Decided on leaving the neighborhood. When we bought this house on Brian Drive there was a lot of hubcaps in the garage and I thought it would make a great decoration in the garage, so cleaned them all and started hanging them on the rafters. Friends would see them and thought I was collecting them, every time they found any, they would give them to me. All the rafters were full, then started from the top down on the walls. Then people began to come looking for a hubcap they might need. I think it was one of the rubbish men that was the first to get a pair he needed. Needless to say, he told his friends. We let them have what they wanted, then they would supply us with more. When it came time for us to move and we didn't know what to do with them somebody said, "You could take them to a car show and sell them." He gave us an idea of their value, so decided to try it. While at one of the car shows with the hubcaps, I saw a set up with pictures of cars to sell. I got the idea of taking old ads from magazines. I would get a roll of Mylar, take cardboard, put the ad on and enclose with mylar. As time went on the ads grew into quite a business. They were outdoing the hubcaps. We sold the hubcap business and went into ads only. This was quite time consuming, but certainly helped to keep your mind busy and not thinking about the cancer. It's bad to let your mind dwell on the thought that you have the cancer. So this was kind of therapeutic, and helped our income. It's great for a person with cancer to have a hobby or something to occupy their mind. In my case it was Bible study, it can become very fascinating and answer a lot of questions about life. Before leaving this, I have one of those stories to tell: We would travel a car show series that took us to Florida, usually for the month of Nov. This provided us with the funds to make it to the next car show. The shows are only on the weekends, so we would need enough to carry us through the week, but one time we had a slight problem. The story follows:We were on our way to Jensen Beach and the finances were very low. The flier we read said this car show started on Friday but arriving then, found out that Friday was for a meeting only. Our finances were down to about $5.00. Upon hearing this news we knew we were in trouble. We asked of any hotel was associated with this car show, as there is usually one. In this particular case it was a Radisson. We went over and asked about the rates. They said, "$75.00 a night." I said, "What is it if you are with the car show?" She said, "$35.00." Then she asked, "Did you want a room or suite?" I said, "What's the difference?" She said, "They're both the same price," so we took the suite. Next she said, "Do you wish to pay now?" We said, "No, when we leave." It came with a continental breakfast. That night we spent our last $5.00 on hot dogs and coffee. This was a two-day show and we were committed to three nights, so we were already in debt before we started. But it turned out to be a very good show and we had enough to pay our bills and move on to the next. At this time we had no credit cards or money in our checking account to fall back on. God is good! We don't know what the future holds, but we know Who holds the future.

Now for another interesting Florida car show story. The first time we went to Daytona for the Turkey Rod Run Show, we stayed at a motel on Daytona Beach and while out for a walk went by a place called "Ocean East". It was lunchtime and the marquis said it had a very good lunch special, so in we went. In the lunch area overlooking the ocean, we picked a table with a beautiful view. At first we just sat there, looking out and thinking how great life is, when the waitress came over and said she could see we'd been through something. We told her it was cancer. She said, "Over the years many people with serious health problems would come and sit there." We told her when she wasn't busy we'd tell her more. Then we began to look around the room and noticed pictures everywhere of people. They were all patrons of the restaurant. When she came back we told her our story, she told us to send her a picture of us because she thought our story would be a great inspiration to others. She displayed our picture where everyone could see it. We still keep in touch. She is one of those beautiful people who you would really love to meet.

Now back to our moving away. We had been out looking for a lot or a home. We thought Canandaigua would be a nice area but found it too expensive for our pocketbook. So as we were driving around we found ourselves in Shortsville. We talked to the realtor. We told him we would like a place near water. He showed us a couple of lots but we didn't like any of them. He took us over on the Canandaigua outlet and showed us another

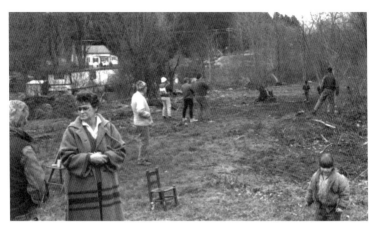

The first picture of the lot to show how much work was involved.

lot in which I was interested. I asked the price but he said his father owned the lot and hadn't decided to sell it yet. He said he'd talk to him. A couple weeks later his mother called and said they'd sell it. This transaction was done the old way-no paper work, just a handshake to seal the deal. A couple weeks later, someone else wanted to buy the property, money on the spot. But the owner said,"No, my handshake is worth more than that money." What a breath of fresh air in this day and age. At the time we purchased this lot, all our friends said it would be too big a job to handle. It probably took 5-600 loads of fill dirt to fill in. We first filled it enough to get our mobile home in and water from the creek would flow into our backyard. There were a lot of huge boulders in the back lot. We got a bulldozer operator to push them over to the bank of the creek. Then we filled it in. The mobile home is 20 feet away from the bank and it's a gorgeous view. Another benefit of this spot was right across the road-a beautiful waterfalls and just this side of the waterfalls was a starting point for the wild water derby. It's white water rafting. What a lot of fun to watch the races right from your own yard. We used to have wonderful garage sales. We now have some mallards we've raised. A lot of fun to watch. Mary and I love it here. It was not a real nice lot and no one could see what it could become, except me. It required a lot of work but turned out to be a beautiful spot.

*Chapter Seventeen*

# Pink Cadillac

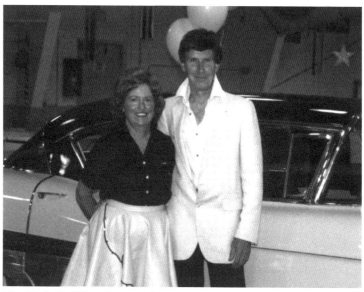

The Pink Cadillac sharing the spotlight with Mary and Ted.

Now we'll go back to the 1957 Cadillac. We took it in to get a paint job. It had already been stripped back to bare metal but fiberglass filled in the spots which were all taken out and metal welded in. An off and on job of two years finally was ready to be painted pink and black and it took until Sept. 16. The Cadillac came out of the paint shop directly to Minett Hall, displayed for the party. That night Cancer Action had a 50's party as it was written in the news ad "Blast from the Past" at the Dome Arena's Minett Hall, from 6 p.m. to midnight. It included fashions and music from the 50's with Big Wheely and the Hubcaps, a hula-hoop contest and a parade of cars. Mary and I were dressed in coordinating outfits. I wore black slacks, a pink shirt and a white sport coat with a pink carnation. Mary wore a pink poodle skirt and a black blouse.

Sometime back when all my hair fell out the doctors gave me a prescription for a wig which I obtained and wore when my hair was all gone. I went into the doctor's office one day and he said, "With all this treatment how come your hair hasn't fallen out?" I just laughed and said, "Can't you tell a wig?" He said, "No, I really couldn't."

Now to get back to the wig and the party. I thought I'd have a good time and see how many I could fool. My wife went with the kids and she didn't know I got out the wig, went to the barber shop and had him put it on to make sure it was all set. Then I went to the party. I walked by my wife and children without them recognizing me. I did it a second time to my wife and on the third time I revealed who I was.

A great time was had by all.

We had our car painted at Fetzner's. It is mostly all brothers who worked there from the Fetzner family. Three of the boys did a lot of work on the car. A week and a half later we took the three boys and their wives out for ice cream. There was a total of eight in the car and nobody was sitting on anybody's lap. After ice cream we stopped back at their shop. We played "Pink Cadillac" with three different versions on cassette coming out through the grill of the car. Then opened up the trunk where we had some hula-hoops left over from "Blast from the Past" party. We played with them in every way except as a hula-hoop. We were having a great time until the cops showed up. It seems we didn't realize we were disturbing the neighborhood.

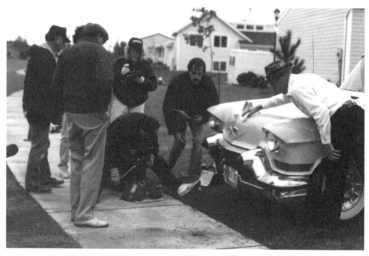

Trying to keep a clean machine, when it was a movie star.

In October '88, through Cancer Action, it had been five years since being diagnosed with two months to live, we got involved with the United Way. While interviewing us they noticed our very positive upbeat attitude. Their campaigns had always been a crying time. This time they decided to go with an upbeat and a more positive film. At this point we were chosen to be part of the film. We were also on a radio commercial. One person we met later had heard it every morning on his way to work and he said that it was so soothing to him. Filming began one week later. The first day of shooting was done at our daughter Tammy's house. Her living room was full of people and equipment. But on Oct. 19 the real star of this whole set up was our '57 pink and black

Cadillac as it rolled into history. Everywhere we had speaking engagements the first question was about that Cadillac. Not how I'm doing, but how's the Cadillac doing. While filming the Cadillac we had a scene where the car came around a curve and the timing was critical. So a man was put in the back seat with earphones and a mike. They would tell him when they wanted the car to come and he would tell me and say how fast to go. It was raining out. This particular shot took five or six takes. At the end of the shooting for the day, I went back to the house and picked up my son and son-in-law to ride with me to take it back to storage. A very funny thing happened on the way, at least it is now. As I'm driving down the road, a police car shows up in my rearview mirror with his candy machine lights on. When I saw this, I said, "He can't want me." I wasn't speeding or doing anything wrong. But he stayed there. I thought he wanted to pass, so I pulled over a little to let him by, but still found he was on my tail. I thought to myself he just wanted to make some comment on the car so I pulled over chuckling to myself. I see him in the mirror getting out of his car and the first thing he did was loosen the flap on his gun, then in a crouched position started approaching my car. I said to the two boys this guy is playing this right to the hilt and we all laughed as we thought this whole thing was a joke. I started to open the door, but he said, "Stay in the car." He put his hand on his gun. I still was looking at the humor in this. So he said, "Roll down the window." I still see he's in a crouched position with hand on his gun. I said, "What's this all about?" "Be quiet, I'll ask the questions." "Where you going?" "Where have you been?" And I said, "What's this all about?" Got no answer. I said, "I'm coming from a filming, the car's in a movie," and "I'm taking it back to storage." He looked in the back seat and said, "Where's the filming equipment?" I said this is a big car but not big enough for all their equipment. The crew that did it came in a furniture van and a couple cars. They went a different way. He asked a few more questions and began to mellow. So I ventured to ask him again, "What's this all about?" He said, "There had been a report on a very suspicious car in one of the neighborhoods." Because it kept circling around the people thought we were casing the homes. I laughed and said to him, "Do you think a crook would be so stupid as to use a '57 pink and black Cadillac to case a place." Give me a break. I knew he was melting because he began to laugh at that. One of the joys having one of those old cars ended well.

After explaining the filming we need to back up and let you know why it was done at our daughter's. We had sold our house in Chili and were staying with her family while our property in Shortsville was being made ready to move in, which happened Dec. 24, 1988. So that's how we wound up in Shortsville. Actually in a little settlement outside of Shortsville, called Littleville, and it's the best Littleville by a dam site. This happened to be Christmas Eve and we had to make a run to 1000 Island Park, to pick up Mary's dad to spend the winter. He was doing winters with us since 1982, as his wife passed on in winter of 1981. We came back to Shortsville the same day; the next day being Christmas. We had to move out of our motel room where we had been staying until our home was ready. We needed to be here on the lot every day, so rented a room in Canandaigua.

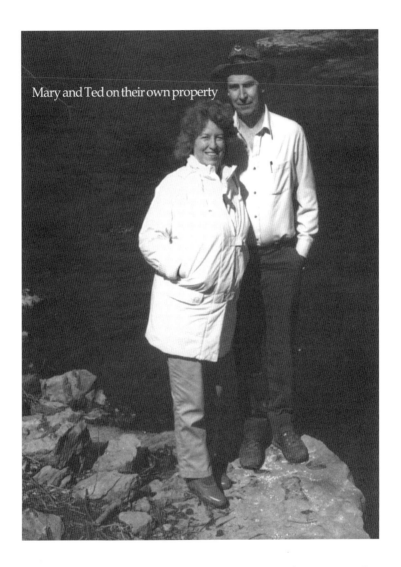
Mary and Ted on their own property

Now out to Littleville. We live on the Canandaigua outlet which is a beautiful spot. It certainly wasn't when we purchased it but that story you've already heard. Right across the road is a beautiful waterfalls. Cancer Action wanted to do a film on us so we told them to visit us and we'd have it done by the falls. It was a beautiful backdrop. It was done Jan. 23, 1989. We never knew anything about the film after it was done, like where it would be shown. But we found out in a funny way. The video was playing at Kodak and our daughter Tammy was working there at the time. She didn't know anything about it so when she spotted it playing she did a double take when she saw her parents. The girl showing the film looked up and saw the expression on her face. She said, "An awful lot of people have fallen in love with the beauty of the waterfalls in the background."

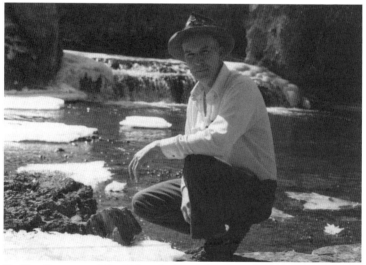

Ted by the water falls. Taken by David Delany for GM Input.
The same spot that was on the Cancer Action film.

Tammy said, "No, no, it's not the waterfalls; that's my parents standing there."

This might be a good time to tell how we got

started with Cancer Action. When I was first diagnosed I was looking for the survivors because all you ever heard was how "Uncle George" died from cancer and how sister and brother passed on. I've heard enough about the people who died. I wanted to find someone I could talk with who was a survivor. Now that it's my turn I know why the survivors don't discuss it. It's very painful because you have to relive it every time you talk about it. I vowed to God if I was a survivor I would talk about it. In the beginning there were many tears shed doing it. I still do it today, although it's difficult, it's not as bad as it was. As I can see the help it provides for others, which makes me feel better about the whole thing. I still work at Cancer Action as a counselor.

Back to the United Way film. We went to a reception on Mar. 7th honoring the stars of the '89 film. This was the first time seeing how the film came out and I first got hooked on their strawberries dipped in chocolate. Man, were they good! We thought it was very well done. On Mar. 10th someone from Rochester Products came to our home for an interview. He took pictures of us by the falls and wrote an article that was put in their paper called "Input".

While going through the United Way we were asked to speak at various companies. Kodak was one of the first. I had worked at Kodak many years prior. I was working at Lincoln Plant when a big government contract got cancelled and quite a few of us were laid off. Because of being a prior employee they wanted me to be there. It was strange being back in an area where I once worked. This was at Elmgrove. When it was over they presented us with a gift of a photo album.

At one of the United Way luncheons I was asked

to drive my Cadillac across the stage. Of course it wasn't the real one it was a cardboard cut out painted like the original. It helped bring a laugh to a very serious luncheon. It was great. I don't want to bore you with all the speaking engagements and luncheons. But I have one more interesting one.

Although I left Rochester Products after the cancer was found, they asked me to speak for the United Way campaign on April 17, 1989 at the Redman's Club. They thought it would be a nice touch for me to bring my granddaughter, Crystal, who was my great inspiration. It turned out to be quite a story. Her mother sent a note to her teacher to let her know she wouldn't be in school the morning of April 17 as she had a breakfast with her Pa for the United Way. I picked her up from her home and took her with us. We had a nice breakfast. During this time we noticed Crystal became very antsy. We didn't know why, she normally didn't act this way. Later we found it was the Chicken Pox. After breakfast I got up to speak and then introduced Crystal as my great inspiration. She ran up and I held her in my arms. What a wonderful way to finish with tears flowing. When she got back to school she had a substitute teacher; the teacher that gave her permission was out. The substitute asked, where she'd been that morning. She just replied, "I went to breakfast with my Nana and Pa." Needless to say the substitute teacher didn't think that was a very good excuse. Of course she didn't know it was for the United Way.

Because of the United Way film the Cadillac drew a lot of interest. So we were asked to participate in a lot of parades and functions. One of them was to start a run at RIT. We actually ran the race for a while. They all thought it was a cool thing to have the car in the lead. We were also asked to participate in the Lilac Parade and I was at Cancer Action talking about this parade when Flora Berg's husband asked what I was wearing. I said I had a black suit and a pink shirt but needed a lilac colored one. He just happened to have a lilac tuxedo shirt with the ruffles. I looked like one sharp dude in that parade. I had the grandchildren in the back seat throwing out candy to the children on the parade route. We were in the Labor Day Parade and got about three blocks into it before the old Cadillac decided she had enough and couldn't be persuaded to go any farther. It was rather embarrassing to push it out of the way.

We've been sharing a lot of fun stuff when all the time I was suffering with the side effects from the treatments and lots of doctor appointments. But throughout this book we want you to know there are two sides to the story. We did all we could to maintain a normal life and not dwell on the bad side of it all. We want you to know we did not just skate free and the other side of the story is the fun things we did through it all.

The first time we were involved with Camp Open Arms was in July 1990. Camp Open Arms is an outreach of Cancer Action. It is a two week camp for children with cancer and their siblings. There is also another cancer camp called Camp Good Days where kids can go away. The kids of Camp Open Arms vacation closer to doctors as they are not as well or have too many appointments. Ours was also a little bit different in that Cobbles School in Penfield was opened up for two weeks to accommodate this camping. The children went home every night by school buses. They would also take us all to Seabreeze for one whole day of a lot of fun. These kids always looked forward to this trip. Some other trips included a tour of the city of Rochester, the Fire Dept. a Donut Shop, etc. We were involved for three years 1990 - 1992. It's a heart breaker but it certainly gave you a wonderful feeling every night when you realized what you had done for those children. You gave them a day to feel normal. We had met some wonderful children. Our group was in the age span of 3-6 year olds. Each of us would be assigned to a different child. They tried to keep it basically a one on one. There were boxes of toys donated for them to play with on a rainy day. In the nice weather they were outside on the swings and slides and they also had small wading pools and sprinklers to run through. We remember one little girl that Mary had whose name was also Mary. You really develop a very close friendship with the one you're assigned to. The minute they see you from the bus in the morning they come looking for you. This little Mary required a painful shot and if she knew it was coming she would run. Mary had to take her for this shot one time and believed it hurt her more than the little girl. It was very painful to have to do this. The next morning she didn't come running to Mary. But the following morning she did come running and what a joy.

Another year Mary and I each had a boy between five and six. The counselors came to us on the day we went to Seabreeze and said that one of the boys had lost a very close friend and would we try to get these two to become friends. We did just that. During the day they went on rides together and down the water slides and had a great time. On the bus going back to school, one of the boys turned to the other one and said, "Will you be my friend?" and he said this to the one that just lost his friend. His reply was, "I don't know, I just lost my last three friends." This is from the mouth of a five year old. What a struggle it must be for the parents of these children.

We won't leave this on the down side but that is just one of the facts.

We have one day when the clowns come. What a wonderful time to watch the kids' faces, when they see the clowns making different animals out of balloons. The clowns would paint their faces. The excitement was fantastic. When the magician came in one day this was quite a sight to see. Everyone was trying to get a front row seat. I think they wanted to see how the tricks were done. On another day the policeman with the talking car came. The kids would follow it trying to find out what made it talk. Then one day a puppet show came and there was another fight for front row seats. These kids were inquisitive. It's a fast-paced two weeks as there's so much that those children want to do, like it's the only two weeks out of the year that they get to live like little children. When you talk with them it's like talking to miniature adults because they have seen so much in such a short span of their lives. We were blessed to have the opportunity to be a part of their life. Like Tiny Tim would say, "God bless us, everyone."

## Chapter Eighteen

# A Milestone
# and Onward

We have finally arrived at 1993 ten years from being told that I had two months to live. It takes ten years before the doctors think you'll make it. What a great feeling to arrive at this great milestone. Just another marker along the way. Cancer is like being on a trip with no final destination until you pass on. There's no time down here that you can say, "I'm free from it." But we go on. We thank God for each new day, as it is a fresh new start, given to you by God so make every day count.

In August while at my brother's town-wide garage sale in Adams my wife took the grandson Bobby to Wellesley Island to visit her father, Chancy Patterson. He lived with us winters and spent summers at his home. She found him not feeling well and did not know that this was the last time she would see him at his home. The next month he was admitted to the hospital in Watertown with stomach cancer. Two weeks later he arrived at our home after we got the 1000 Islands Park Ambulance to transport him. Within two days our neighbor had a large car to transport him to Genesee Hospital. We were in the hospital visiting Mary's dad. The other guy in his room was carrying on and making all kinds of funny noises while we were there but Chancy, even though he was so sick, told us just to ignore him, he couldn't help himself. What a statement for him to make. How many people would think that way? Instead they would complain to the nurse. But this quiet, gentle talking 89 year old man made the statement, "He can't help himself." Take this as your thought for today. He was there for three weeks. Then came back to our home in October and lived his time at our home where he passed on Jan. 7, 1994. It's an awful hard thing to watch a very close family member slowly slip away and leave you. But we know where he went. As Mary's mother came to us one day and said she was not sure whether Chancy was a born-again Christian or not. She said, "He went forward once but didn't think it was for God, but to just make me happy." For us to make sure that he was, when he was in the hospital, we asked Pastor Ray Drake to visit him and make sure of his salvation. He in turn told us that he had done so. When he told him to confess he was a sinner he started confessing everything right there and the Pastor heard more than he really wanted to know.

This would be a good spot to go back and let you know that, while going through the cancer ordeal we were taking care of my mom with Alzheimer's and Mary's dad, Chancy. Mom's care was split between myself and my younger brother Bob and his family. Bob's family liked to be able to celebrate the holidays so we took her for the winters and he took her for the summers, and it worked out well. Occasionally we would go there and take her to the 1000 Islands. She was born in the same house in Clayton, as well as her mother and grandmother. So she had a love also for the river and watching the big boats, even in her advanced stage of Alzheimer's. You could see her face light up to watch the ships go by. It was a labor of love taking care of the two. She passed on Nov. 1987. We were all determined that we wouldn't let them fall into the hands of a nursing home.

But before we leave the parents, we have a couple funny stories that shouldn't get left out.

One night Mary, I, Grampa and my mom were doing a puzzle and eating ice cream. My mom started mumbling, we looked and she was putting puzzle pieces on her ice cream. The reason for the mumble-she had put some in her mouth. We had to immediately remove them before she choked on them. Now we can look back and laugh, but at that time it was not a laughing matter.

After a TOPS Meeting (Take off pounds sensibly) we were at a restaurant with all the girls and they knew my mom had Alzheimer's. Also, strange and funny things do happen. On this particular day Chancy was with us. This happens to be one of the funniest. We were sitting there after our orders were in, all of a sudden my mom reached in her purse for something wrapped in toilet paper. Not looking too pretty. She handed it to me and said, "These are yours." So I took the gooey mess out of her hand, with all eyes on me, I opened it, and in total surprise, it was a set of false teeth. We could not imagine where they came from. She said they were mine, but I knew differently as I had mine in place. So figured they were hers, until a small voice from the other end of the table says, "They are mine." It was Mary's dad, Chancy. They were Chancy's and he was very embarrassed, as he was a very proud man, and having this happen in front of all these women was no picnic for him.

When you're around someone with Alzheimer's

disease, don't think that they're dumb because they can't remember names or stupid because they don't talk. Don't ever think that they don't have feelings. This is a story on feelings that will break your heart. My mother hadn't spoken in a year and a half and didn't know us for the last two years. She went to bed one night and had a bad case of the runs during the night. When we got around in the morning, we found her laying in this awful mess. We had to cut her nightgown from her and pick her up out of it, get her to the bathroom and into the tub. Mary even had to wash her hair, as everything was a mess. Got some clean clothes on her and we proceeded to leave the bathroom. At the door mom grabbed Mary. Mary couldn't imagine what was happening. Mom wanted to give Mary a big hug, and said "Thank you!" She hadn't spoken before and she didn't again. She managed to express her feelings at that time, which proves that their feelings are still there. It's just difficult for them to express it.

Now, after filling you in with all that, we'll get back to our topic, cancer.

I'm seeing Doctor Asbury and Doctor Schneider at least once a year at this time. I have brought up my lack of energy but nobody thought too much about it until I went to a speaking engagement and lost my train of thought. I started to cry and just couldn't remember anything and had to leave the platform. I was also having trouble with my neck, it was always stiff, etc. This is all from the treatments. Turns out I had an underactive thyroid. This is caused by the whole brain radiation that was given and I'm told that with an overactive thyroid they use radiation to bring it down. But mine was good so the radiation brought it down further.

I did not know how much an underactive thyroid affected me but Friday and Saturday when they changed that medication they wanted it done instantly so to speak. They called the prescription into Fay's Drugs and I went in to pick it up. When I got there I asked the pharmacist what an underactive thyroid did and she said it affected everything in the body - the heart, the blood pressure, all your vital organs, the muscles. You will have trouble with your neck and it leaves you tired all the time.

You know I can go to bed and sleep 8-10 hours and wake up just like I haven't been to bed yet. And that's just the way I feel. Even now I feel like I'm about half here. It'll make you short of wind and give you trouble getting around. There's a whole lot of stuff to it. Now they are finally getting concerned. And they've been working on it to bring it back into balance. They'll just allow it to go higher and higher until they get to the point where it stops. So, instead of going for a year, they're having me come in every couple of months.

## Story of Faith

We were at a church sale and they knew they would have a great deal of clothing left over. They wanted to know if we could take it where it would be of benefit. We said, "Yes, we had been thinking, it would be a nice trip to take stuff to the Appalachians, as we heard there were a lot of poor families there." So we went to the library and got a book on the Appalachians to locate the poorest areas. We found one and went to AAA and made out our trip tik for VA. The next day we had to pick up the clothes. When we arrived they were putting them in boxes. I told them not to as boxes would take up too much room. We had our 1994 Buick wagon and they stated we couldn't get them all in. I said, "Stand back and watch." We got them all in. They said, "We have a box of stuffed animals we don't know what to do with." I said, "That's all right I'll put them in." I lined them up in the back windows along the sides and across the back all facing out the windows. What a sight to see. All these animals looking out as we drove down the road. That night God told us to go to a city on the border of Virginia and Kentucky. So, as you might guess, time to get a new trip tik. On our trip down, we saw places looking for donations and Mary thought we should stop to drop off our stuff as it would make the trip quicker. Let me state here that with all this stuff we had we had no idea of where it would wind up or what was happening. But I decided we had to go to this city, even though we didn't know where we were going in this city. By the time we arrived we were in this dark strange city not knowing where to go and only one listing by AAA in their book. So we decided that was best but no idea how to get there. We wound up in a shabby part of town when we saw a man and asked him where this motel was. He tried to explain the directions, but we were all confused and he said, "Follow me, and I'll take you there." He had a pretty rough car, but very happy to do us the favor. After we arrived there I offered him a $5.00 bill for gas, and he turned it down but I made him take it. He was just one of those wonderful people you meet now and then.

Now we're at the motel and we went to check in. While checking in the clerk said, "Are you here for business or pleasure?" We said, "We're here on God's business." She wanted to know what we meant. So we said, "We have a carload of clothes and stuffed animals for the needy." But we didn't know where we were going with them. This is about 11:00 p.m. She said, "I'll send someone down to your room to talk to you." So around midnight there was a knock on the door. We soon found out it was the clerk's husband who just happened to be a Baptist minister in charge of clothing distribution for seven counties and he had three churches. It kept him running on Sunday morning to tend to all three. It took 60 miles to accomplish. But he said, "Tomorrow a.m. be at my house for breakfast." This was in Kentucky. We had a wonderful breakfast and fellowship! Then off to work. In order for him to ride with us, we had to empty the back seat, so they got black garbage bags and filled them with clothes and put them in their small pick-up. Just to get it so we had the back seat we filled their little pick-up with the clothes. This gives you an idea of how tightly packed the car was. They were stacked floor to ceiling with no air pockets. The stuffed animals were still lined up; waiting in the back of the wagon still packed with clothes. We took off, and got to one of the poor areas and stopped for coffee and pie. When we came out we found the wagon encircled with children looking at all those stuffed animals. It was quite a sight to see. I went over and told each child to pick out one. This was like watching kids in a candy store trying to pick out the best one. As they picked their favorite I would reach in and hand out the one they chose. What a wonderful sight to see the happy expressions of love on their faces as they wrapped their arms around their choice. After leaving we went to one of his churches and he called a couple of ladies to come over and start sorting out the rest of these clothes and animals. It took a while to unload everything. Then the Pastor invited us to stay for Sunday, the next day, at his house so we could attend one of his churches. On the way to his church he asked if I would speak for about 10 minutes. So after the singing he introduced me and I went up to the pulpit and started talking. I took up all his time for the whole service. Every time I looked his way he was smiling. After leaving the service we started home with our mission fully accomplished leaving us with a beautiful memory.

Now to close out the book we're going back to the beginning to the diner where we used to meet Peg Leg in PA. One day near the end of our book writing we were in downtown Rochester heading for the AAA office. While waiting for a light where I was going to turn I got this overwhelming urge to go straight which took me into the Strong Museum parking lot. Not knowing why I was there I said, "Let's go into the museum." I walked through the front door and there in front of me was a complete diner. It said Skyliner over it and I said, "Mary, we've been there before. That diner looks familiar." So we decided to go in for lunch and once inside I knew I'd been in this diner before but couldn't place where so we asked the waitress and she said, "It was from PA." and I said, "That's it, this is Mountain Top Diner," and she said, "Yes, it is." We could almost feel Peg Leg sitting with us. The story of the diner goes like this:

It was built in New Jersey and it was moved to about 10 miles north of Williamsport, Pa. on Rt. 15. George Hiras was the original owner and he operated the Mountain Top Diner until 1991 when it had to be moved because of a new road. It was bought by a couple in Rochester who owned the Highland Diner. They couldn't get the city's approval to set it up so they wound up selling it to the Strong Museum where it still operates today and they renamed it Skyliner. What a wonderful way to end with a place to go that takes you back to the beginning of the story where we first came in contact with cancer. It's like a memorial to our friend, Peg Leg. God is so good.

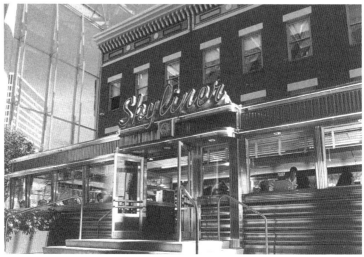

What a surprise, when we found it again at Strong Museum, where we can go and relive our memories.

### A footnote to this whole story:

As far as we know, before me there were no survivors, and since there have been no survivors as of 2001, I have no idea why God picked me to live but it was all done in His hands. You should get to know Him.

### A note from Ted:

In this book I have mentioned my medications for information only, because now they would be changed. But God never changes, he always remains the same. If you are going through cancer, you should ask him to go with you.

## ACKNOWLEDGEMENTS

Most of all I have to thank God for saving my life.

Next I want to thank my wife who stood by me through it all.

Without the encouragement of Ted Williams, and his guidance to the end, this book would not have made it from our mind and on to paper.

Without our daughter, Tammy Cook, none of the writing part of it would have been done. She had the patience to help us rewrite this book, at least five times.

Thank you Linda Coe for a wonderful job of editing and guiding us with this book.

Also Morry Barkley for putting it in to the computer.

I want to thank my brother, Bob Cornell, for taking the photo for the cover.

I would also like to thank Larry Cultrera for the use of his photo of the Mountain Top Diner.

Strong Museum now has Mountain Top Diner and they call it Sky Liner. Thanks for the information.

I want to also acknowledge Drs. Asbury, Sobel and Craver and thank them for their help and support.

Last but not least, thanks to David Delaney of Gm Input for the beautiful pictures bythe creek.

'For I know the plans that I have for you', declares the Lord, 'plans for welfare and not for calamity to give you a future and hope. (Jeremiah 29:11)
Ted and Mary are living testimonies to God's faithfullness. This book reveals their walk of faith through the shadowy valley trusting in God's word. May your heart be stirred as you travel these pages with them.

*Linda Coe*

There is no doubt in our mind that you have managed to make the best of your life, because of the Love for each other "In Christ". It is encouraging to see the wisdom in living as you are alive and not as you are going to die. You didn't let the adversary "steal your joy" and proved that fervent prayers prevail. You didn't let the heartaches keep you down showing that there is hope out there for people to have loving marriages and a special relationship with God.

I know that you Ted, through Christ conquered other obstacles like quitting habitual drinking and smoking earlier in life. (Mary you proved that faith the size of a mustard seed would move a mountain.) People truly suffer from these habits and search their whole lives for the peace and joy. I hope that through this testimony people will find courage to put their trust in God and meet Jesus as he stands at the door of their heart.

May you continue to be blessed with wisdom and abounding joy for living your life fully in Christ Jesus!

Bill and Carolyn DeLong

This book is an amazing account of God's ways. Relationships, losses and pain are just the background to Ted's life; a living miracle of serving, believing and walking in the joy of the lord. Throughout the whole healing experience in God's hands, Ted Cornell's were toward the Lord. My faith was definitely challenged.

Sue Markus

# Cancer Is So Limited

It cannot cripple Love
It cannot shatter Hope
It cannot corrode Faith
It cannot destroy Peace
It cannot kill Friendship
It cannot invade the Soul
It cannot silence Courage
It cannot steal Eternal Life
It cannot conquer the Spirit
It cannot suppress Memories

Author unknown

Eze 30:21 Son of man, I have broken the arm of Pharaoh king of Egypt; and, lo, it shall not be bound up to be **healed**, to put a roller to bind it, to make it strong to hold the sword.

Eze 34:4 The diseased have ye not strengthened, neither have ye **healed** that which was sick, neither have ye bound up [that which was] broken, neither have ye brought again that which was driven away, neither have ye sought that which was lost; but with force and with cruelty have ye ruled them.

Eze 47:8 Then said he unto me, These waters issue out toward the east country, and go down into the desert, and go into the sea: [which being] brought forth into the sea, the waters shall be **healed**.

Eze 47:9 And it shall come to pass, [that] every thing that liveth, which moveth, whithersoever the rivers shall come, shall live: and there shall be a very great multitude of fish, because these waters shall come thither: for they shall be **healed**; and every thing shall live whither the river cometh.

Eze 47:11 But the miry places thereof and the marishes thereof shall not be **healed**; they shall be given to salt.

Hsa 7:1 When I would have **healed** Israel, then the iniquity of Ephraim was discovered, and the wickedness of Samaria: for they commit falsehood; and the thief cometh in, [and] the troop of robbers spoileth without.

Hsa 11:3 I taught Ephraim also to go, taking them by their arms; but they knew not that I **healed** them.

Mat 4:24 And his fame went throughout all Syria: and they brought unto him all sick people that were taken with divers diseases and torments, and those which were possessed with devils, and those which were lunatick, and those that had the palsy; and he **healed** them.

Mat 8:8 The centurion answered and said, Lord, I am not worthy that thou shouldest come under my roof: but speak the word only, and my servant shall be **healed**.

Mat 8:13 And Jesus said unto the centurion, Go thy way; and as thou hast believed, [so] be it done unto thee. And his servant was **healed** in the selfsame hour.

Mat 8:16 When the even was come, they brought unto him many that were possessed with devils: and he cast out the spirits with [his] word, and **healed** all that were sick:

Mat 12:15 But when Jesus knew [it], he withdrew himself from thence: and great multitudes followed him, and he **healed** them all;

Mat 12:22 Then was brought unto him one possessed with a devil, blind, and dumb: and he **healed** him, insomuch that the blind and dumb both spake and saw.

Mat 14:14 And Jesus went forth, and saw a great multitude, and was moved with compassion toward them, and he **healed** their sick.

Mat 15:30 And great multitudes came unto him, having with them [those that were] lame, blind, dumb, maimed, and many others, and cast them down at Jesus' feet; and he **healed** them:

Mat 19:2 And great multitudes followed him; and he **healed** them there.

Mat 21:14 And the blind and the lame came to him in the temple; and he **healed** them.

Mar 1:34 And he **healed** many that were sick of divers diseases, and cast out many devils; and suffered not the devils to speak, because they knew him.

Mar 3:10 For he had **healed** many; insomuch that they pressed upon him for to touch him, as many as had plagues.

Mar 5:23 And besought him greatly, saying, My little daughter lieth at the point of death: [I pray thee], come and lay thy hands on her, that she may be **healed**; and she shall live.

Mar 5:29 And straightway the fountain of her blood was dried up; and she felt in [her] body that she was **healed** of that plague.

Mar 6:5 And he could there do no mighty work, save that he laid his hands upon a few sick folk, and **healed** [them].

Mar 6:13 And they cast out many devils, and anointed with oil many that were sick, and **healed** [them].

Luk 4:40 Now when the sun was setting, all they that had any sick with divers diseases brought them unto him; and he laid his hands on every one of them, and **healed** them.

Luk 5:15 But so much the more went there a fame abroad of him: and great multitudes came together to hear, and to be **healed** by him of their infirmities.

| |
|---|
| *healed* occurs **79** times in **77** verses: Page 3, verses 51 - 75 |
| Luk 6:17 And he came down with them, and stood in the plain, and the company of his disciples, and a great multitude of people out of all Judaea and Jerusalem, and from the sea coast of Tyre and Sidon, which came to hear him, and to be **healed** of their diseases; |
| Luk 6:18 And they that were vexed with unclean spirits: and they were **healed**. |
| Luk 6:19 And the whole multitude sought to touch him: for there went virtue out of him, and **healed** [them] all. |
| Luk 7:7 Wherefore neither thought I myself worthy to come unto thee: but say in a word, and my servant shall be **healed**. |
| Luk 8:2 And certain women, which had been **healed** of evil spirits and infirmities, Mary called Magdalene, out of whom went seven devils, |
| Luk 8:36 They also which saw [it] told them by what means he that was possessed of the devils was **healed**. |
| Luk 8:43 And a woman having an issue of blood twelve years, which had spent all her living upon physicians, neither could be **healed** of any, |
| Luk 8:47 And when the woman saw that she was not hid, she came trembling, and falling down before him, she declared unto him before all the people for what cause she had touched him, and how she was **healed** immediately. |
| Luk 9:11 And the people, when they knew [it], followed him: and he received them, and spake unto them of the kingdom of God, and **healed** them that had need of healing. |
| Luk 9:42 And as he was yet a coming, the devil threw him down, and tare [him]. And Jesus rebuked the unclean spirit, and **healed** the child, and delivered him again to his father. |
| Luk 13:14 And the ruler of the synagogue answered with indignation, because that Jesus had **healed** on the sabbath day, and said unto the people, There are six days in which men ought to work: in them therefore come and be **healed**, and not on the sabbath day. |
| Luk 14:4 And they held their peace. And he took [him], and **healed** him, and let him go; |
| Luk 17:15 And one of them, when he saw that he was **healed**, turned back, and with a loud voice glorified God, |
| Luk 22:51 And Jesus answered and said, Suffer ye thus far. And he touched his ear, and **healed** him. |
| Jhn 5:13 And he that was **healed** wist not who it was: for Jesus had conveyed himself |

away, a multitude being in [that] place.

Act 3:11 And as the lame man which was **healed** held Peter and John, all the people ran together unto them in the porch that is called Solomon's, greatly wondering.

Act 4:14 And beholding the man which was **healed** standing with them, they could say nothing against it.

Act 5:16 There came also a multitude [out] of the cities round about unto Jerusalem, bringing sick folks, and them which were vexed with unclean spirits: and they were **healed** every one.

Act 8:7 For unclean spirits, crying with loud voice, came out of many that were possessed [with them]: and many taken with palsies, and that were lame, were **healed**.

Act 14:9 The same heard Paul speak: who stedfastly beholding him, and perceiving that he had faith to be **healed**,

Act 28:8 And it came to pass, that the father of Publius lay sick of a fever and of a bloody flux: to whom Paul entered in, and prayed, and laid his hands on him, and **healed** him.

Act 28:9 So when this was done, others also, which had diseases in the island, came, and were **healed**:

Hbr 12:13 And make straight paths for your feet, lest that which is lame be turned out of the way; but let it rather be **healed**.

Jam 5:16 Confess [your] faults one to another, and pray one for another, that ye may be **healed**. The effectual fervent prayer of a righteous man availeth much.

1Pe 2:24 Who his own self bare our sins in his own body on the tree, that we, being dead to sins, should live unto righteousness: by whose stripes ye were **healed**.

You are on page 3 of 4. To view other pages, select page number. (Verse range also shown)

*healing* occurs **14** times in **13** verses:

Jer 14:19 Hast thou utterly rejected Judah? hath thy soul lothed Zion? why hast thou smitten us, and [there is] no **healing** for us? we looked for peace, and [there is] no good; and for the time of **healing**, and behold trouble!

Jer 30:13 [There is] none to plead thy cause, that thou mayest be bound up: thou hast no **healing** medicines.

Nah 3:19 [There is] no **healing** of thy bruise; thy wound is grievous: all that hear the bruit of thee shall clap the hands over thee: for upon whom hath not thy wickedness passed continually?

Mal 4:2 But unto you that fear my name shall the Sun of righteousness arise with **healing** in his wings; and ye shall go forth, and grow up as calves of the stall.

Mat 4:23 And Jesus went about all Galilee, teaching in their synagogues, and preaching the gospel of the kingdom, and **healing** all manner of sickness and all manner of disease among the people.

Mat 9:35 And Jesus went about all the cities and villages, teaching in their synagogues, and preaching the gospel of the kingdom, and **healing** every sickness and every disease among the people.

Luk 9:6 And they departed, and went through the towns, preaching the gospel, and **healing** every where.

Luk 9:11 And the people, when they knew [it], followed him: and he received them, and spake unto them of the kingdom of God, and healed them that had need of **healing**.

Act 4:22 For the man was above forty years old, on whom this miracle of **healing** was shewed.

Act 10:38 How God anointed Jesus of Nazareth with the Holy Ghost and with power: who went about doing good, and **healing** all that were oppressed of the devil; for God was with him.

1Cr 12:9 To another faith by the same Spirit; to another the gifts of **healing** by the same Spirit;

1Cr 12:30 Have all the gifts of **healing**? do all speak with tongues? do all interpret?

Rev 22:2 In the midst of the street of it, and on either side of the river, [was there] the tree of life, which bare twelve [manner of] fruits, [and] yielded her fruit every month: and the leaves of the tree [were] for the **healing** of the nations.